Women's He

T0229179

Editors

HEATHER P. ADAMS
ALEECE R. FOSNIGHT

PHYSICIAN ASSISTANT CLINICS

www.physicianassistant.theclinics.com

Consulting Editor
JAMES A. VAN RHEE

July 2018 • Volume 3 • Number 3

ELSEVIER

1600 John F. Kennedy Boulevard • Suite 1800 • Philadelphia, Pennsylvania, 19103-2899

http://www.theclinics.com

PHYSICIAN ASSISTANT CLINICS Volume 3, Number 3
July 2018 ISSN 2405-7991, ISBN-13: 978-0-323-61315-6

Editor: Jessica McCool
Developmental Editor: Casey Potter

Physician Assistant Clinics (ISSN: 2405–7991) is published quarterly by Elsevier Inc., 360 Park Avenue South, New York, NY 10010-1710. Months of issue are January, April, July, and October. Periodicals postage paid at New York, NY and additional mailing offices. Subscription prices are $150.00 per year (US individuals), $205.00 (US institutions), $100.00 (US students), $150.00 (Canadian individuals), $257.00 (Canadian institutions), $100.00 (Canadian students), $150.00 (international individuals), $257.00 (international institutions), and $100.00 (international students). Foreign air speed delivery is included in all *Clinics* subscription prices. All prices are subject to change without notice. POSTMASTER: Send address changes to *Physician Assistant Clinics*, Elsevier Periodicals Customer Service, 11830 Westline Industrial Drive, St. Louis, MO 63146. Customer Service Health Sciences Division, Subscription Customer Service, 3251 Riverport Lane, Maryland Heights, MO 63043. **Customer Service: 1-800-654-2452 (U.S. and Canada); 314-447-8871 (outside U.S. and Canada). Fax: 314-447-8029. E-mail: journalscustomerservice-usa@elsevier.com (for print support); journalsonlinesupport-usa@elsevier.com (for online support).**

Reprints. For copies of 100 or more, of articles in this publication, please contact the Commercial Reprints Department, Elsevier Inc., 360 Park Avenue South, New York, NY 10010-1710. Tel. 212-633-3874; Fax: 212-633-3820; E-mail: reprints@elsevier.com.

Physician Assistant Clinics is covered in *EMBASE/Excerpta Medica and ESCI*.

PROGRAM OBJECTIVE

The goal of the *Physician Assistant Clinics* is to keep practicing physician assistants up to date with current clinical practice by providing timely articles reviewing the state of the art in patient care.

TARGET AUDIENCE

Physician Assistants and other healthcare professionals.

LEARNING OBJECTIVES

Upon completion of this activity, participants will be able to:
1. Review polycystic ovarian syndrome and benign breast disease
2. Discuss the clinical approach to diagnosis and management of recurrent pregnancy loss.
3. Recognize components of the female athlete triad.

ACCREDITATION

The Elsevier Office of Continuing Medical Education (EOCME) is accredited by the Accreditation Council for Continuing Medical Education (ACCME) to provide continuing medical education for physicians.

The EOCME designates this enduring material for a maximum of 15 *AMA PRA Category 1 Credit*(s)™. Physicians should claim only the credit commensurate with the extent of their participation in the activity.

All other health care professionals requesting continuing education credit for this enduring material will be issued a certificate of participation.

DISCLOSURE OF CONFLICTS OF INTEREST

The EOCME assesses conflict of interest with its instructors, faculty, planners, and other individuals who are in a position to control the content of CME activities. All relevant conflicts of interest that are identified are thoroughly vetted by EOCME for fair balance, scientific objectivity, and patient care recommendations. EOCME is committed to providing its learners with CME activities that promote improvements or quality in healthcare and not a specific proprietary business or a commercial interest.

The planning committee, staff, authors and editors listed below have identified no financial relationships or relationships to products or devices they or their spouse/life partner have with commercial interest related to the content of this CME activity:
Heather P. Adams, MPAS, PA-C; Stevi Barrett, MMS, PA-C; Meredith Browne, MMS, PA-C; Linda Burdette, MPAS, PA-C; Joseph Daniel; Emily S. Edmondson, MPAS, PA-C; Emily S. Edmondson, MPAS, PA-C; Stephanie P. Elko, MSPAS, PA-C; Tiffany Esinhart, MMS, PA-C; Aleece Fosnight, MPAS, PA-C, CSC, CSE; Deborah A. French, MSPAS, PA-C, MT (ASCP); Rebecca Gimpert, MMS, PA-C; Laura Icenhour, MMS, PA-C; Casey Potter; Alison Kemp; Sarah Lindahl, PA-C; Erin McCartney, MPAS, PA-C; Jessica McCool; Kristen M. Murphy, PT, DPT; Caroline Palmer, MPAS, PA-C; Carla Picardo, MD, MPH; Suzanne Reich, MPAS, PA-C; Natalie Richard, MPAS, PA-C; Tiffany Riley, MPAS, PA-C; Elyse Watkins, DHSc, PA-C.

The planning committee, staff, authors and editors listed below have identified financial relationships or relationships to products or devices they or their spouse/life partner have with commercial interest related to the content of this CME activity:
Nisha McKenzie, PA-C, CSC, IF: has served on a speaker's bureau for AMAG Pharmaceuticals, Inc.
James A. Van Rhee, MS, PA-C: receives royalties and/or holds patents from Kaplan, Inc.

UNAPPROVED/OFF-LABEL USE DISCLOSURE

The EOCME requires CME faculty to disclose to the participants:
1. When products or procedures being discussed are off-label, unlabelled, experimental, and/or investigational (not US Food and Drug Administration [FDA] approved); and
2. Any limitations on the information presented, such as data that are preliminary or that represent ongoing research, interim analyses, and/or unsupported opinions. Faculty may discuss information about pharmaceutical agents that is outside of FDA-approved labelling. This information is intended solely for CME and is not intended to promote off-label use of these medications. If you have any questions, contact the medical affairs department of the manufacturer for the most recent prescribing information.

TO ENROLL

The CME program is available to all *Physician Assistant Clinics* subscribers at no additional fee. To subscribe to the *Physician Assistant Clinics*, call customer service at 1-800-654-2452 or sign up online at www.physicianassistant.theclinics.com.

METHOD OF PARTICIPATION

In order to claim credit, participants must complete the following:

1. Complete enrolment as indicated above.
2. Read the activity.
3. Complete the CME Test and Evaluation. Participants must achieve a score of 70% on the test. All CME Tests and Evaluations must be completed online.

CME INQUIRIES/SPECIAL NEEDS

For all CME inquiries or special needs, please contact elsevierCME@elsevier.com.

Contributors

CONSULTING EDITOR

JAMES A. VAN RHEE, MS, PA-C
Associate Professor, Program Director, Yale School of Medicine, Yale Physician Assistant Online Program, New Haven, Connecticut

EDITORS

HEATHER P. ADAMS, MPAS, PA-C
Associate Professor, Physician Assistant Department, Gannon University, Clinical Physician Assistant, Women's Wellness and Gynecology, Erie, Pennsylvania

ALEECE FOSNIGHT, MPAS, PA-C, CSC, CSE
Clinical Physician Assistant, Pisgah Urology, Transylvania Regional Hospital, Transylvania County Department of Public Health, AASECT Certified Sexuality Counselor and Educator, Mission Medical Associates, Brevard, North Carolina; Founder, Southeastern Sexual Health Society, Asheville, North Carolina

AUTHORS

HEATHER P. ADAMS, MPAS, PA-C
Associate Professor, Physician Assistant Department, Gannon University, Clinical Physician Assistant, Women's Wellness and Gynecology, Erie, Pennsylvania

STEVI BARRETT, MMS, PA-C
Gastroenterology, Digestive Health Specialists, Clemmons, North Carolina

MEREDITH BROWNE, MMS, PA-C
Obstetrics and Gynecology, Wake Forest Baptist Medical Center, Winston-Salem, North Carolina

LINDA BURDETTE, MPAS, PA-C
Clinician, Premier Women's Health of Yakima, Yakima, Washington

EMILY S. EDMONDSON, MPAS, PA-C
Physician Assistant, Vineyard Primary Care, UPMC Hamot, North East, Pennsylvania

STEPHANIE P. ELKO, MSPAS, PA-C
Director of Clinical Education, Physician Assistant Studies, Assistant Professor, Augsburg University, Minneapolis, Minnesota

TIFFANY ESINHART, MMS, PA-C
Emergency Medicine, US Acute Care Solutions, Carolinas Healthcare System, Charlotte, North Carolina

ALEECE FOSNIGHT, MPAS, PA-C, CSC, CSE
Clinical Physician Assistant, Pisgah Urology, Transylvania Regional Hospital, Transylvania County Department of Public Health, AASECT Certified Sexuality Counselor and Educator, Mission Medical Associates, Brevard, North Carolina; Founder, Southeastern Sexual Health Society, Asheville, North Carolina

DEBORAH A. FRENCH, MSPAS, PA-C, MT (ASCP)
Physician Assistant Studies Volunteer Faculty, Volunteer and Community Faculty, Practicing as a PA-C Advanced Internal Medicine, University of Kentucky, West Paducah, Kentucky

REBECCA GIMPERT, MMS, PA-C
Hospital Medicine, Carolinas Hospitalist Group, Carolinas Healthcare System, Charlotte, North Carolina

LAURA ICENHOUR, MMS, PA-C
Emergency Medicine, US Acute Care Solutions, Carolinas Healthcare System, Charlotte, North Carolina

SARAH LINDAHL, PA-C
Sutter East Bay Medical Foundation, Castro Valley, California

ERIN McCARTNEY, MPAS, PA-C
Division of Maternal Fetal Medicine, Eastern Virginia Medical School, Norfolk, Virginia

NISHA McKENZIE, PA-C, CSC, IF
Physician Assistant, Women's Health, Center for Women's Sexual Health, Grand Rapids OB/GYN, Grand Rapids, Michigan

KRISTEN M. MURPHY, PT, DPT
Pelvic Health Physical Therapist and Clinical Director, Perfect Balance Physical Therapy, Brevard, North Carolina

CAROLINE PALMER, MPAS, PA-C
Assistant Professor, Physician Assistant Department, Gannon University, Erie, Pennsylvania

CARLA PICARDO, MD, MPH
Owner and Clinically Practicing Obstetrician/Gynecologist, Women's Wellness and Gynecology, Erie, Pennsylvania; Clinical Assistant Professor of Obstetrics, Gynecology, and Reproductive Sciences, The University of Pittsburgh School of Medicine, Pittsburgh, Pennsylvania

SUZANNE REICH, MPAS, PA-C
Associate Professor, Program Director, Department of PA Studies, Wake Forest School of Medicine, Winston-Salem, North Carolina

NATALIE RICHARD, MPAS, PA-C
Cardiothoracic Surgery Residency Program, UPMC Presbyterian, Pittsburgh, Pennsylvania

TIFFANY RILEY, MPAS, PA-C
Physician Assistant, Shepard Creek OB/GYN, Farmington, Utah

ELYSE WATKINS, DHSc, PA-C
Assistant Professor, Department of Physician Assistant Studies, High Point University, High Point, North Carolina

Contents

Three distinct entities comprise what is known as the female athlete triad: low energy availability, menstrual dysfunction, and diminished bone mineral density. If there is caloric restriction, many of the body's metabolic and neuroendocrine processes shut down, leading to a state of oligomenorrhea or amenorrhea, which is most often the first recognizable presentation. There is a disruption in the hypothalamus pituitary gonadal axis. Losing bone mass may increase fracture risk and sets the stage for early-onset osteoporosis caused by the associated hormonal imbalance. The cornerstone of treatment involves education and intervention from a multidisciplinary team.

This article discusses the physician assistant (PA) role in sexuality counseling and the importance of recognizing sexual health as part of the overall health and well-being of female patients. There is discussion on the prevalence of sexuality concerns, models for sexuality counseling, implementation of brief sexual symptom checklist, and specific suggestions that the PA can recommend to increase the satisfaction of sexual functioning.

Long-acting reversible contraceptives (LARCs), the intrauterine device and implant, are recommended as the first line of contraception by the American College of Obstetrics and Gynecology and the American Academy of Pediatrics for adolescents in the United States because of their low failure rate and high compliance, but the United States has high teen pregnancy rates. Barriers to more prevalent use include patient and provider misconceptions regarding infection, infertility, and insertion. Overall, the risk of adverse outcomes with LARC use is low and fertility is maintained after removal. Addressing misconceptions will lead to increased use of LARCs and decreased unintended pregnancies.

Polycystic ovarian syndrome (PCOS) is one of the most common metabolic disorders of premenopausal women. In patients with PCOS, multiple systems are affected: reproductive, metabolic, dermatologic, and psychological. Although the cause and pathogenesis of this condition are not entirely understood, the acknowledgment of PCOS for more than 80 years in the medical community has resulted in developing techniques to treat the symptoms to improve the quality of life for patients who suffer from this condition. PCOS is accompanied by other medical complications, but with management by the patient's health care team, a promising prognosis is possible.

Benign breast disease is a common finding in women and is an important risk factor for future breast cancer. Benign lesions may be nonproliferative, proliferative without atypia, or proliferative with atypia. Lesions include breast cysts, fibroadenomas, intraductal papillomas, and hyperplasia. Diagnostic imaging and biopsy are required for definitive diagnosis, and excision may be necessary depending on the histology of the lesion.

The average life expectancy for an American woman is 81 years. As such, she spends nearly one-third of her life in postmenopause. If a woman experiences a bilateral oophorectomy before menopause, the ratio naturally increases. Long-term physiologic effects of menopause, primarily caused by estrogen deficiency, are separated into two broad categories: effects on the brain and effects on the body. Since the initiation of the Women's Health Initiative in 1991, research identified new opportunities for treating the neurocognitive, emotional, and somatic effects of menopause. PAs should be aware of current guidelines regarding screening and treating the common issues associated with menopause.

Low libido is the most common sexual problem facing women. Female sexual interest and arousal disorder is vastly underrecognized in the medical community. This article highlights screening options, current diagnostic criteria, prevalence, as well as treatment and counseling options.

Pregnant women infected with human immunodeficiency virus (HIV) are at risk for perinatal HIV transmission from mother to fetus. The first step in perinatal transmission reduction is the identification of HIV during pregnancy, followed by antiretroviral therapy (ART). ART is effective at reducing perinatal transmission if started, ideally prepartum, and the woman has good ART response. When choosing ART, providers must take into account multiple factors, including an understanding of the HIV replication cycle, patient perinatal status (antepartum, intrapartum, or postpartum), patient ART status (treatment naive, previous therapy, and current therapy), and patient response to ART, mode of delivery, and timing of delivery.

Challenging Vaginas: Case Studies in Recognizing and Treating Vulvovaginitis

Linda Burdette

Bacterial vaginosis, vulvovaginal candidiasis, and trichomoniasis are the most common causes of vaginitis in premenopausal women. Vulvovaginal atrophy is the most common cause of vulvovaginal discomfort in postmenopausal women. This article consists of various case studies that look at the diagnostic presentation of these common disorders, treatment options for recurrent or chronic vulvovaginitis, and finally a look at less common causes of vulvovaginitis.

A Review of Infertility for the Primary Care Provider

Sarah Lindahl

Infertility and subfertility are common phenomena in health care. The causes of infertility vary widely, do not necessarily remain constant throughout a couple's relationship or an individual's lifetime, and can be multifactorial, all of which add to the challenge of diagnosing and treating infertility. A multitude of infertility evaluation strategies and techniques are used by primary care providers, including physician assistants. A solid understanding of the causes, diagnostic techniques, and management strategies for infertility and subfertility allows primary care providers to provide and/or facilitate the care of these patients.

Centering Pregnancy: A Novel Approach to Prenatal Care

Heather P. Adams and Carla Picardo

Centering Pregnancy offers the traditional components of prenatal care along with patient education and development of a support system through use of a group health care model. The approach of a health care provider promotes patient empowerment and a sense of control over her own health and that of her fetus. Evidence suggests improved obstetric, reproductive, and public health outcomes for patients who participate in Centering Pregnancy. Implementation and growth of new programs have challenges, and Centering Pregnancy is no exception; however, the benefits of this program should provide ample motivation to overcome challenges for the benefit and satisfaction of patients.

The Role of Pelvic Floor Physical Therapy for the Female Patient

Kristen M. Murphy and Aleece Fosnight

This article imparts to the medical providers a better understanding of the function and role of the pelvic health physical therapist in the treatment of

Recurrent pregnancy loss (RPL) affects 1% to 5% of couples trying to conceive, who often feel frustrated and desperate for answers. RPL has classically been defined as loss of 3 pregnancies before 20 weeks' gestation. With the American Society for Reproductive Medicine guidelines, it is reasonable to begin evaluation and management after 2 consecutive pregnancy losses. With conflicting evidence in the literature, it is a challenge for clinicians to determine the best path for diagnosing and treating patients with RPL. This article reviews currently accepted diagnosis and management, discusses controversial treatments available, and gives guidance on the diagnosis and treatment of RPL.

PHYSICIAN ASSISTANT CLINICS

THE CLINICS ARE AVAILABLE ONLINE!
Access your subscription at:
www.theclinics.com

Foreword
Women's Health

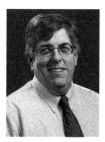

James A. Van Rhee, MS, PA-C
Consulting Editor

In 2015, Dr Flavia Bustreo, Assistant Director General for Family, Women's and Children's Health through the Life-Course, World Health Organization, discussed the top ten main issues regarding women's health that keep her up at night.[1] The top ten list included the following:

- Cancer
- Reproductive health
- Maternal health
- HIV
- Sexually transmitted infections
- Violence against women
- Mental health
- Noncommunicable diseases
- Being young
- Getting older

While we cannot cover all these topics in this issue of *Physician Assistant Clinics*, we have covered a number of the topics. Reproductive health issues and maternal health issues are responsible for many of the health issues for women between the ages of 15 and 44 years. In this area, Lindahl reviews infertility; Adams and Picardo review prenatal care; French discusses recurrent pregnancy loss; and Fosnight covers sexuality counseling. As HIV infection rate is rapidly growing in young women, Eiko and McCartney discuss pregnancy and HIV. The rates of sexually transmitted diseases continue to increase, and more now than ever, education in regards to prevention and treatment is so important. Also, Burdette covers the diagnosis and treatment of vulvovaginitis. In the area of getting older, we have Watkins discussing menopause and Fosnight and Murphy discussing the role of physical therapy in pelvic floor disorders. Noncommunicable diseases account for millions of deaths per year in women.

Physician Assist Clin 3 (2018) xiii–xiv
https://doi.org/10.1016/j.cpha.2018.04.002
2405-7991/18/© 2018 Published by Elsevier Inc.

physicianassistant.theclinics.com

Richard, Palmer, and Adams discuss the female athlete triad; Browne, Barrett, Icenhour, Reich, Gimpert and Esinhart discuss the barriers to the use of long-acting reversible contraceptives in adolescents. Other topics in this issue include McKenzie, who discusses female sexual interest and arousal disorder; Edmondson, who reviews polycystic ovarian syndrome; and Riley, who reviews benign breast diseases. As you can see, a wide variety of articles.

A special thanks to Heather Adams from Gannon University and Aleece Fosnight from Transylvania Regional Hospital, both also from the Association of PAs in OB/Gyn, who served as guest editors for this issue. I hope you enjoy this issue of *Physician Assistant Clinics*. Our next issue will provide you with a review of the latest in geriatrics.

James A. Van Rhee, MS, PA-C
Yale School of Medicine
Yale Physician Assistant Online Program
100 Church Street South, Suite A230
New Haven, CT 06519, USA

E-mail address:
james.vanrhee@yale.edu

Website:
http://www.paonline.yale.edu

REFERENCE

1. World Health Organization. Ten top issues for women's health. 2015. Available at: http://www.who.int/life-course/news/2015-intl-womens-day/en/. Accessed March 21, 2018.

Preface

Promoting the Role of Physician Assistants in Women's Health

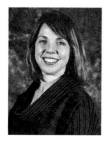 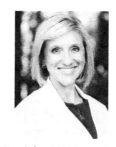

Heather P. Adams, MPAS, PA-C   Aleece Fosnight, MPAS, PA-C, CSC, CSE
Editors

As PAs who have dedicated the majority of our years in clinical practice to women's health, we are honored to contribute to an issue of *Physician Assistant Clinics* that highlights the area of medicine that we are passionate about. As active members serving on the board of the Association of Physician Assistants in Obstetrics and Gynecology (APAOG), we find ourselves working alongside the other leaders of APAOG looking for ways to advocate for the PA role in women's health care with the common goal of improving women's access to the highest quality of care that exists. The *Physician Assistant Clinics'* focus on the delivery of "authoritative and continuously updated clinical information," written "for PAs by PAs," further promotes the role of PAs in all facets of women's health care.

This issue includes a wide breadth and depth of women's health topics, written from the perspective of practicing PAs and other health care providers who work closely with PAs. In this issue, you encounter topics relating to high-risk obstetrics, innovations in prenatal care, challenges and barriers to health care, sexual health, female athletes, acute and chronic gynecologic pathologic conditions, promising treatment strategies, breast health, menopause, and female adolescent health. These works represent the expertise, sacrifice, and passion of each of our valued authors. These women are truly leaders in our field, and we feel *blessed/honored/privileged* to call them colleagues and friends. We are excited to offer you a detailed look into these fascinating topics, and as you read this special issue of the *Physician Assistant Clinics*, we hope for the following:

- That your knowledge base expands and your horizons are broadened
- That you find yourself asking questions and continuing the lifelong learning process

Physician Assist Clin 3 (2018) xv–xvi
https://doi.org/10.1016/j.cpha.2018.04.001
2405-7991/18/© 2018 Published by Elsevier Inc.

- That you gain enthusiasm for the instrumental role that PAs can, and do, play in caring for women of all walks of life and that you feel challenged to find your own role as an advocate for PAs in women's health!

Heather P. Adams, MPAS, PA-C
Physician Assistant Department
Gannon University
109 University Square
Erie, PA 16541, USA

Women's Wellness and Gynecology
Erie, PA 16506, USA

Aleece Fosnight, MPAS, PA-C, CSC, CSE
Pisgah Urology
Transylvania Regional Hospital
87 Medical Park Drive, Suite A
Brevard, NC 28712, USA

Southeastern Sexual Health Society
Asheville, NC, USA

E-mail addresses:
adams051@gannon.edu (H.P. Adams)
aleece.fosnight@gmail.com (A. Fosnight)

Female Athlete Triad
Low Energy Availability, Menstrual Dysfunction, Altered Bone Mineral Density

Natalie Richard, MPAS, PA-C[a,1], Caroline Palmer, MPAS, PA-C[b,*,2],
Heather P. Adams, MPAS, PA-C[c]

KEYWORDS

• Female athlete triad • Anorexia • Amenorrhea • Osteoporosis

KEY POINTS

• The female athlete triad (FAT) consists of 3 components: low energy availability, menstrual dysfunction, and decreased bone mineral density.
• Those most at risk include those involved in esthetically pleasing sports that emphasize low body weight.
• Restricting calories, whether purposeful or unintentional, causes the body to conserve energy by altering metabolism and neuroendocrine pathways.
• Because of the many possible factors that contribute to low energy availability, treatment of individuals presenting with 1 or more of the components of the FAT may require intervention of a multidisciplinary team.
• Education on appropriate nutrition and calorie consumption for female athletes is a key component of prevention because low energy availability is the primary driving factor of the triad.

INTRODUCTION

Female participation in sports is often associated with many physiologic, sociologic, and psychological benefits. However, the development of the female athlete triad (FAT) may have an alarming effect on the overall health and development of physically

Disclosure: Each author does not have any relationships with a commercial company that has a direct financial interest in the subject matter or materials discussed in the article or with a company making a competing product.
[a] Department of Cardiothoracic Surgery, UPMC Presbyterian, Suite C800, 200 Lothrop Street, Pittsburgh, PA 15213, USA; [b] Physician Assistant Department, Gannon University, 109 University Square, Erie, PA 16541-0001, USA; [c] Physician Assistant Department, Gannon University, 109 University Square, Erie, PA 16541, USA
[1] Present address: 338 Browns Mill Road, Evans City, PA 16033.
[2] Present address: 913 Cherry Hill Boulevard, Erie, PA 16509.
* Corresponding author.
E-mail address: palmer018@gannon.edu

Physician Assist Clin 3 (2018) 313–324
https://doi.org/10.1016/j.cpha.2018.02.001
2405-7991/18/© 2018 Elsevier Inc. All rights reserved.

physicianassistant.theclinics.com

active women, which extends beyond their level of performance on the field. The FAT consists of 3 distinct interrelated conditions: low energy availability, menstrual dysfunction, and altered bone mineral density (BMD).[1–10] The components of the FAT should be viewed on a spectrum varying from normal function to dysfunction. This spectrum allows for a broader and less rigid view of presenting symptoms that makes for an easier diagnosis and earlier treatment plan. The 3 components can occur on a sliding scale that may occur at different rates in accordance with the athlete's diet and exercise habits.[7,9]

EPIDEMIOLOGY

The FAT is most commonly seen in female athletes competing in sports or activities that emphasize low body weight. Gymnastics, cross-country running, ballet dancing, figure skating, and swimming are a few examples, with gymnastics being the most common. Often, athletes are under intense stress to maintain a lean body mass to better enhance their athletic performance.[1,5,6,9,10] However, in doing so, female athletes may find themselves performing below their peak level because of the associated conditions that play a part in the FAT. It is often manifested under specific conditions; the high desire to improve athletic performance, a win-at-all-costs mentality, and coach/parents' negligence in adequately recognizing the signs that make up the FAT.[9]

CAUSE

A study published in the *Medicine & Science in Sports & Exercise* reported that the prevalence of 2 components of the triad was between 3% and 27% and the expression of any single component was 16% to 60%, indicating that most athletes only present with 1 or 2 of the 3 components of the triad.[4,7,10,11] Another study received from the *Archives of Pediatric and Adolescent Medicine* revealed that, out of 170 high school female athletes, 18.3% met the criteria for disordered eating, 23.5% for menstrual irregularity, and 21.8% for low bone mass. However, of these athletes, only 5.9% presented with 2 components and 1.2% presented with all 3.[12]

Low Energy Availability

Exercising extreme weight control for the sake of performance and aesthetic purposes is a common feature in physically active women. Energy availability is expressed as the total dietary energy in calories (calories in) minus the total exercise energy expended (calories out), or the amount of energy that remains in the body that is available for sports performance.[4,7,9] Low energy availability is considered to be the driving force and cornerstone of the triad and may be the result of either decreased caloric intake or increased output.[4,7,9,10] In any case in which an athlete intensifies her workload during training, she also needs to increase her caloric intake as well to protect against any energy imbalance.[4,7,10]

In the short term, an athlete may have decreased strength, power, and stamina caused by an energy deficiency from failure to maintain proper food fueling with carbohydrates and protein intake or inadequate stores.[7,10] In a study published in the *Journal of Sports Science* involving female collegiate soccer players (a sport usually not associated with disordered eating), up to one-third of the team displayed low energy availability (<30 kcal/kg) over the course of the season.[13]

Low energy availability is not synonymous with disordered eating in that most cases occur without an eating disorder.[4,7,9,10] Some athletes are unaware, or lack the nutritional knowledge, that the amount of calories expended during exercise is not replaced by their total dietary intake.[7] A study published in the *International Journal of Sports Physical Therapy* investigated 89 female athletes competing in interscholastic cross-country and track. This study revealed that only a small percentage of runners with an associated musculoskeletal injury reported disordered eating behaviors and attitudes. This finding may suggest that these young adolescent girls may be unaware of the energy intake level needed to support their high energy expenditure. However, the possibility must be considered that athletes did not respond truthfully to the initial eating disorder screening survey (EDE-Q) out of belief that thinness leads to an increased performance.[6] Otherwise, low energy availability may also occur secondary to an eating disorder such as anorexia nervosa or bulimia.[4,7,9,14] Consequences are inevitable, because the energy required for proper physiologic functioning is not available.[7]

An article titled, "Nutritional Practices Associated with Low Energy Availability in Division I Female Soccer Players" followed 19 collegiate soccer players throughout the fall competitive season with the purpose of examining the macronutrient intake, energy density, and intake distribution related to low energy availability. The American College of Sports Medicine (ACSM) recommendations for carbohydrate intake during the preseason and midseason were not met in 73% of participating athletes. Another finding revealed that many of the participating athletes were reluctant to eat a well-balanced wholesome dinner following a soccer game. Making conscientious strides to restrict calories in order to maintain a low body weight may serve as a possible explanation for this conveyed observation. Those engaging in this purposeful behavior of choosing low-energy-density foods may do so in spite of body dissatisfaction and drive for thinness.[15]

Menstrual Dysfunction

The prevalence of menstrual dysfunction in many young female athletes may be as high as 79%.[4] Menstrual dysfunction is manifested as irregular cycles or progress to amenorrhea. Most severe is amenorrhea, which may be subcategorized in 2 different types: primary amenorrhea and secondary amenorrhea. The FAT could cause either type. Identification of true dysfunction in young female athletes also proves to be difficult to detect because 65% of girls show signs of oligomenorrhea during their first year after menarche.[7] Strenuous training alone may not be the only factor in causing abnormalities in a woman's menstrual cycle because dietary restriction may also be a contributing factor.[4,9] To maintain eumenorrhea, women need to consume approximately 45 kcal/kg fat-free mass (FFM) per day. Oligomenorrhea typically occurs in women consuming less than 30 kcal/kg FFM per day.[3,9] Therefore, special attention should be paid to the diet of female athletes partaking in vigorous exercise before menarche.

Low Bone Mineral Density

When comparing athletes with nonathletes, athletes typically display a BMD that is higher than that of the average nonathlete, especially in athletes participating in any weight-bearing sport.[4,7,9,10,14] The most critical time frame for bone growth for women is within the 2 years following menarche, with bone development reaching its peak by 20 to 25 years of age.[7,10] Impaired bone growth during this age range is concerning and could lead to a greater risk of developing osteoporosis in the future.[4,7–10] Decreased BMD with menstrual irregularities also puts athletes at a greater risk for fractures, particularly stress fractures.[6,10] Stress fractures of the tibia account for 25% to 63% of all stress fractures in female athletes.[9,10]

Referring to a study published in the *International Journal of Sports Physical Therapy* regarding 89 high school cross-country athletes, the most frequent site of injury occurred in the lower leg (shin/calf), making up 46.2% of all injuries.[6] All athletes participating in the study underwent a BMD measurement of the spine, proximal femur, and tibia/fibula, as well as an entire body dual-energy x-ray absorptiometry (DEXA) scan. Runners with low BMD were found to be at a 5-fold to 6-fold increased risk of injury.[6] The current study's results determined that runners who reported oligomenorrhea/amenorrhea within the past year and low BMD according to their associated age range correlated with an increase in lower extremity musculoskeletal injuries.[6]

PHYSIOLOGY

The physiology of the hypothalamic-pituitary-ovarian axis relies on pulsatile release of gonadotropin-releasing hormone (GnRH) from the hypothalamus, which in turn stimulates follicle-stimulating hormone (FSH) and luteinizing hormone (LH) from the anterior pituitary. FSH-stimulated follicular development occurs in the early part of the menstrual cycle, leading to follicular development. LH-stimulated ovulation forms a dominant follicle signaling the beginning of the luteal phase. The area of ovulation then develops into the corpus luteum. Both the developing follicles in the follicular phase and the corpus luteum in the luteal phase secrete estrogen and progesterone (Fig. 1). The level of these hormones has significant impact on the development of the uterine endometrium. Estrogen is dominant in the follicular phase, leading to thickening and stabilization of the uterine endometrium. Progesterone is dominant in the luteal phase, leading to changes in the endometrium in preparation for either implantation of a fertilized ovum or menstruation if fertilization does not occur. Dysfunction in any step of this process could result in decreased follicular development, anovulation, and absence of a corpus luteum, thus affecting the total levels, as well as balance, of estrogen and progesterone. An offset causes an imbalance between these two hormones, thus affecting the development and functionality of the endometrium.[2–5,7,9,10]

Neuroendocrine Dysfunction

Restricting calories, whether purposeful or unintentional, causes the body to conserve energy by altering metabolism and neuroendocrine pathways.[2–5,7,9,10] The type of amenorrhea resulting from energy availability is functional hypothalamic amenorrhea, caused by suppression of the hypothalamic-pituitary-ovarian axis and alteration in its normal functioning, which is described earlier.[10] A suppression at any phase of the axis results in the disruption of the menstrual cycle and circulating hormones.

Women with low levels of circulating estrogen may present with several other features that prove to be detrimental to their overall health. Increased low-density lipoprotein (LDL) levels combined with endothelial dysfunction may result in cardiovascular disease.[2,3] In eumenorrheic athletes, estrogen helps to promote the release of endothelial nitric oxide, which in turn helps to promote several antiatherosclerotic properties such as decreased platelet aggregation, smooth muscle proliferation, and LDL oxidation.[2,9] Because estrogen has a protective effect on bone mass by inhibiting osteoclasts, any deficiency in estrogen creates an environment in which bone may be more susceptible to increased boney turnover rendering early onset osteoporosis.[2–5,7,9] Energy availability less than 30 kcal/kg FFM fails to reach the threshold needed to maintain the pulsatile release of FSH and LH and further reduces bone formation with an increase in bone resorption.[2–5,7,9]

An associated link between fat mass and low energy availability with altered pulsatile GnRH secretion may endure through the production of other neuroendocrine hormones such as adipokines, which have a known impact on the hypothalamus pituitary

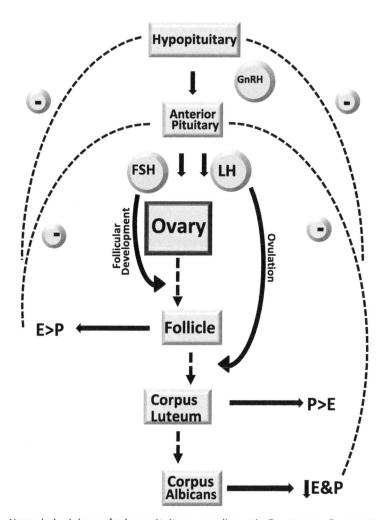

Fig. 1. Normal physiology of a hypopituitary gonadism axis. E, estrogen; P, progesterone.

gonadal axis.[2,4,5] Decreased adipokines, particularly leptin, correlate very strongly with energy deprivation and in disorders associated with low fat mass.[4,5,9] Leptin is an important determinant of pulsatile LH secretion and its deficiency contributes to the loss of menses.[4,5,9]

Not only serving as a measure of energy storage, fat mass is also found to play a role in the disturbance of another set of neuroendocrine hormones: ghrelin, peptide YY (PPY), insulin, cortisol, and growth hormone (GH), with insulinlike growth factor 1 (IGF-1).[2,4,5] Levels of ghrelin reflect overall energy status and are inversely associated with fat mass because decreased calories intake may cause an increased level of ghrelin. High levels of ghrelin may also suppress LH and FSH pulsatility, further impairing the GnRH pituitary axis.[2,4,5] An increased level of PPY has been linked to GnRH suppression, which is commonly seen in female athletes who present with the triad in addition to anorexia nervosa.[2,3,5] Insulin and glucose levels are typically decreased in low energy states. Insulin promotes LH pulse frequency; therefore, a decrease in insulin has a negative effect on LH secretion.[2,4,5] As an adaptive response to maintain euglycemia in amenorrheic athletes, there is an overactivity of the hypothalamic-pituitary-adrenal axis that causes an increase in the amount of cortisol being released.[2,4,5] An increase in the pulsatile GH secretion with an associated decreased IGF-1 suggests an acquired hepatic resistance to GH.[2,5] A summary of all increased and decreased levels is given in **Table 1**.

SCREENING AND DIAGNOSIS

One of the greatest challenges in managing adolescent female athletes is the initial diagnosis of the triad. As recommended by the ACSM, screening for elements of the triad should be conducted at preparticipation physical examinations as well as annual health checkups, especially if the patient presents with triad signs and symptoms.[4,5,7,9,10] Suggested screening tools include the LEAF (Low Energy Availability in Females) Questionnaire, Eating Disorders Inventory (EDI-3), and the EAT-26 to properly assess any patient suspected of having low energy availability.[7] Often, young female athletes are reluctant to confess behaviors that may reveal a fear of weight gain or issues with body image. Because the eating patterns of young physically active women are often obscured and do not qualify as an established diagnosis of anorexia nervosa or bulimia, the subclinical diagnosis of an eating disorder often goes unnoticed, leading to mistreatment.[7]

Any patient who presents with 1 aspect of the triad should be screened for the remaining parameters, because most may present with only 1 but are at risk for all 3.[1,4,7,9,10] Several red flags should be raised in any woman who presents with amenorrhea or recent injury, particularly multiple reoccurring stress fractures. A thorough and detailed history should be obtained, paying particular attention to menstrual status, diet and eating behaviors, physical activity regimen, and past repetitive injuries.[4,7,9,10] In addition, focused questions regarding age of menarche, presence of any psychological stressors, and training intensity with frequency of sport should be asked and may be helpful in determining energy balance in these athletes.[4,7,9,10] A more detailed panel of screening questions for use during a preparticipation examination is listed in **Table 2**.

Physical examination findings suggestive of the triad include signs related to nutritional deficiency and caloric deprivation.[4,9] A complete list of pertinent physical examination findings can be found in **Table 3**. Calculation of a patient's body mass index (BMI) or body fat percentage should also be obtained.[4,7] In the evaluation of primary or secondary amenorrhea, causes such as hypothyroidism/hyperthyroidism, pituitary tumors, polycystic ovarian syndrome, hyperandrogenism, and birth control should be considered as differential diagnoses.[4,10] A list of required diagnostic tests is given in **Table 4** in order to rule out these associated diagnoses.

Table 1 Neuroendocrine alterations in the female athlete triad	
Increased	**Decreased**
Ghrelin	LH and FSH
Cortisol	Estrogen
GH	Leptin
LDL	Peptide YY
	Insulin
	IGF-1

Data from Refs.[2,4,5]

Table 2
Screening questions for the female athlete triad

Question	Red Flags
What sport do you participate in?	Thin-image sports (distance running, dance, gymnastics)
How many hours a day do you train?	Multiple practices a day, year-round practices, an athlete who trains markedly longer than others in the same sport
How do you feel about your body/weight?	Responses like "I'm too fat/skinny", "I'd be faster if I was thinner"
Do you eat breakfast?	Never being hungry for breakfast
What do you eat in a typical day?	Refusal to answer. Choosing only junk or snack food. Vegetarian/vegan. "I never eat___"
Have you started your periods?	No start by age 15 y or started and then stopped
When was your last period?	Cycles >35 d, no periods for 3 mo
Have you even broken a bone? Which one? How?	Any recurrent fractures, stress fractures, fractures with little or no force involved
Do you drink milk? Calcium supplements?	Never, seldom, cannot tolerate

Data from Refs.[4,7,9,10]

According to the ACSM, any female athlete suspected of having the triad who presents with oligomenorrhea/amenorrhea for greater than 6 months, disordered eating, and history of stress fractures should have a bone scan with DEXA.[2–4,7,9,10] The DEXA scan is recognized as the gold standard to measure bone mineral density because of its speed, precision, safety, and low cost.[2–4,7,9,10] Measurement of bone mass in the spine and hip is standard for young women. Because T-scores prove unreliable in premenopausal women, the Z-score of age-matched individuals is predominately

Table 3
Physical examination findings suggestive of the female athlete triad

Examination Component	Findings
Vitals	Low BP or orthostasis, bradycardia, weight/fluctuations or significant weight loss, high or low BMI
General	Anxious, overly thin, paleness, fatigue, arrested growth, delayed puberty, dry hair or hair loss
HEENT	Dental erosions/caries, enlarged parotid glands, dry mucous membranes
Cardiovascular	Sinus bradycardia or other arrhythmias, postural or nonpostural hypotension
Gastrointestinal	Discomfort, full abdomen/constipation, rectal prolapse
Musculoskeletal	Muscle weakness, bone pain, joint pain
Extremities	Edema
Neurologic	Peripheral neuropathy
Skin	Lanugo, hand abrasions, dry skin

Abbreviations: BP, blood pressure; BMI, body mass index; HEENT, head, eyes, ears, nose, and throat.
Data from Refs.[4,7,10]

Table 4
Suggested diagnostic tests in diagnosing the female athlete triad

Tests Conducted in Order to Rule Out an Eating Disorder	Athletes That Present with Amenorrhea
• CBC	• Beta-human chorionic gonadotropin
• CMP	• Thyroid-stimulating hormone
• B_{12}	• Free thyroxine
• Folate	• Prolactin
• Salivary amylase	• FSH and LH hormonal levels
• Creatinine	• Total testosterone
• Glucose	• Sex hormone-binding globulin
• ECG	• Progesterone challenge

Abbreviations: CBC, complete blood count; CMP, complete metabolic panel; ECG, electrocardiogram.
Data from Refs.[3,4,7,10]

used.[3,6] Athletes categorized as having low BMD are 1 or 2 standard deviations less than the age-matched, gender-specific Z-score. Therefore, Z-scores between −1 and −2 should be a cause for concern.[6] **Table 5** summarizes a DEXA scan assessment for an abnormal BMD.

MANAGEMENT WITH A MULTIDISCIPLINARY APPROACH

Because of the many possible factors that contribute to low energy availability, treatment of individuals presenting with 1 or more FAT components may require the intervention of a multidisciplinary team, which may include sports dieticians, athletic trainers, coaches, psychologist, health care providers, and parents.[2–4,7,9,10] It is important that all members of the team collaborate and work together because of an athlete's intricate history and variable presentation, paying specific attention to the psychological burden the triad may have on the individual.[7] Once identified, the cornerstone of treatment is increasing overall energy availability by means of increased caloric intake and reduced caloric expenditure, which helps to achieve the overall treatment goal in reestablishing a menstrual cycle and enhancing bone mineral density.[2–4,7,9,10]

Management of Caloric Deficits

Referral to a registered dietician often is the first step in initiating care and maintaining the athlete's optimal energy availability. An increase of at least 30 to 45 kcals/kg in combination with calcium and vitamin D supplementation is the current recommendation and has been shown to quickly improve BMD in patients with prolonged amenorrhea.[3] Depending on the age of the patient, the duration of the triad, and the time to recovery with the resumption of menses, BMD may stabilize and improve. However, patients may not necessarily return to baseline or even age-appropriate BMD.[10]

Table 5
Assessment of dual-energy x-ray absorptiometry scan with abnormal bone mineral density

BMD Z-Score	Diagnosis
Between −1.0 and −2.0	Low BMD
Les than −2.0	Osteoporosis

Data from Refs.[2–4,6,9,10]

Significant changes in BMD may be observed in as little as 3 months, with further improvement only if healthy weight and adequate nutrition are maintained for the following 12 months.[3,10] Stressing the importance of weight gain of any amount in these patients may help improve bone health and lay the foundation of overall success management.[10]

Management of Psychiatric Implications

One of the greatest barriers in the guidance of young female athletes is the psychological burden that encompasses and drives many of their actions and habits.[10] Treatment may be very difficult and may involve seeking out the assistance of a mental health specialist. This difficulty may arise because female athletes are often competitive, determined individuals with perfectionist personalities, and may carry a fear of changing their (successful in sport-related results) diet and exercise regimens.[10] It is most beneficial to engage in activities that require less energy expenditure, such as cross-training, resistance, or balance training, rather than exercise restriction.[3] Recognition of psychological pressures must be addressed early to ensure timely intervention.[2–4,7,9,10]

Pharmaceutical Management

Although pharmacologic therapies do not play a large role in the treatment of the FAT, hormonal therapies specifically may still be used to help augment nutrition counseling.[2–4,7,9] Combination oral contraceptive pills (OCPs) may be initiated to help a woman return to monthly menses through regular withdrawal bleeding.[3,10] However, the use of combination OCPs does not normalize natural metabolic hormones such as FSH, LH, leptin, ghrelin, IGF-1, GH, and cortisol. The restoring of lost BMD is not supported by the use of combination OCPs and may even cause a premature closure of the epiphyseal growth plate in young female athletes.[3] Misinterpretation of a hormonal withdrawal bleed as a healthy return of a menstrual cycle may cause a false sense of security and subsequently encourage a female patient to remain stable at a weight that may be far less than the treatment goal for full recovery.[3]

Regarding direct treatment of low bone mineral density in premenopausal women, bisphosphonates are contraindicated because of their prolonged half-life and teratogenic effects.[2–4,7,10] Simple weight gain and supplementation with calcium and vitamin D is highly recommended for improvement of BMD.[3] Bone mineral density assessment should be considered if a patient is at high risk for decreased BMD to better cater for a treatment regimen.[3]

PREVENTION

Primary prevention should focus on education. Education about the signs and symptoms of the FAT should be a priority among all health care professionals, coaches, and caregivers involved in the lives of female athletes.[2,4,7,10] An article titled "Female Athlete Triad Awareness Among Multispecialty Physicians" surveyed 931 physician participants (pediatricians, internists, and family medicine physicians) to assess triad knowledge in the health care arena. Overall, 37% had heard of the triad, and of the respondents around 51% reported feeling comfortable treating patients with the triad. One of the roles of physicians and physician assistants is performing the preparticipation sports examinations, working closest with the affected female aged population (12–25 years old). It is reasonable to conclude that they should be most familiar with the triad risks and consequences.[1] Given the low awareness of the triad in the health care community, efforts should be made to integrate the FAT into the curriculum of various health care professions.[1] Physician assistants, trained under a medical model that focuses on primary care, are employed in a wide variety of health care settling and specialties and are well suited to screen for, diagnose, and treat FAT.

Education on appropriate nutrition and calorie consumption for female athletes is a key component of prevention because low energy availability is the primary driving factor of the triad. This education should involve the athlete, the coaches, and parents.[10] Nutrient-dense foods with a low glycemic index should be initiated with a detailed plan of action, mapping out certain foods to help gear the athlete toward a better diet that will adequately meet the caloric demands of the sport. Advising young physically active women to consume the recommended amount of calcium and vitamin D during the adolescent years is essential for proper bone banking and BMD maintenance.[1,6]

One of the greatest barriers to the treatment of young women with the triad is overcoming the psychological component of their condition.[10] Female athletes are often led to believe that to be the best they have to be "skinny" or look a certain way. Along with nutritional education, changing the mindset of female athletes is important regarding prevention of an associated eating disorder.[7,16] An athlete's main support team, composed of coaches, athletic trainers, and parents, must be aware of and able to identify behaviors that predispose athletes to FAT.[16] Even seemingly casual side comments about weight from coaches can precipitate a cascade of unhealthy decisions. An online survey of 227 high school coaches was used to construct a study titled Gender Differences in High School Coaches' Knowledge, Attitudes, and Communication about the female Athlete Triad. Results revealed that significant differences were observed relating to attitudes and communication regarding eating and menstrual irregularity. Male coaches were considerably more likely than female coaches to advise athletes to eliminate certain foods or even skip a meal in order to achieve a perceived body image to enhance sport performance.[16] Similarly, an overwhelming number of male coaches were under the impression that amenorrhea is a normal occurrence in highly trained athletes.[16] In the survey, coaches did express an interest in receiving educational material and strategies to provide a more effective means of communication between coaches and athletes addressing sensitive issues like menstrual irregularity.[16] Coaches play an important role in early detection and must feel comfortable speaking up about any suspicious signs and rigid eating behavior, even if it is occurring simultaneously with personal bests and records. An athlete's coach may be the first to notice any change in the athlete's performance, exercise routine, and behavior and must feel comfortable making the athlete aware of her condition.[4,7] However, referrals to a psychologist may help facilitate a plan of care when there are concerns by an athlete's family or coaching staff.

Specialty programs such as Athletes Targeting Health Exercise and Nutrition Alternatives (ATHENA) have been designed with both a psychological and nutritional component that educates young athletes on self-esteem, societal pressure, and sports nutrition.[7] Clearly, proper screening at preparticipation physical examinations with a detailed and focused history provide the best opportunity to recognize concerning behaviors and allow for early patient education in female patients who may be at risk for development of the triad.[5,7]

SUMMARY

The FAT is a potentially serious condition that is composed of 3 interrelated components: high caloric deficit, menstrual irregularity, and loss of bone mineral density.[1–10] Young female athletes who tend to be the most vulnerable to developing the triad are those competing in sports in which the pressure to be thin may take precedence over making healthy decisions.[1,5,6,9,10] It is crucial that athletes who present with any 1 or 2 of these components be assessed for FAT.[1,10] Because decreased energy availability is the cornerstone of the triad, educating athletes, coaches, parents, and health practitioners about the requirements for optimal energy intake, energy balance, and fuel intake is essential.[1,7,9,10,16] When energy intake is insufficient to meet individual needs, the body is forced to conserve energy by shutting off many of the body's neuroendocrine mechanisms. Most notable is the hypothalamic-pituitary-gonadal axis, in which the body may no longer produce enough estrogen to maintain regular menses, potentially resulting in low BMD.[2,5,7,9,10] The ultimate goal of treatment involves reestablishing a menstrual cycle and enhancing BMD primarily through increasing energy availability.[7] A multidisciplinary team approach to management proves to be the most successful approach to achieve the goals of prevention of FAT as well as appropriate management of the complexity of the triad.[2–4,7,9,10]

REFERENCES

1. Curry EJ, Logan C, Ackerman K, et al. Female athlete triad awareness among multispecialty physicians. Sports Med Open 2015;1(1):38. Available at: https://www.ncbi.nlm.nih.gov/pmc/articles/PMC4642583. Accessed July 15, 2016.
2. Barrack MT, Ackerman KE, Gibbs JC. Update on the female athlete triad. Curr Rev Musculoskelet Med 2013;6(2):195–204. Available at: https://www.ncbi.nlm.nih.gov/pmc/articles/PMC3702770. Accessed July 15, 2016.
3. Kansdorf L, Vegunta S, Files J. Everything in moderation: what the female athlete triad teaches us about energy balance. J Womens Health 2013;22(9):790–2. Available at: https://www.ncbi.nlm.nih.gov/pubmed/22741211. Accessed July 15, 2016.
4. Payne J, Kirchner J. Should you suspect the female athlete triad? J Fam Pract 2014; 63(4):187–92. Available at: https://www.ncbi.nlm.nih.gov/pubmed/24905120. Accessed July 15, 2016.
5. Mira M. Neuroendocrine mechanisms in athletes. Handb Clin Neurol 2014;124: 373–86. Available at: https://www.ncbi.nlm.nih.gov/pubmed/25248600. Accessed July 15, 2016.
6. Rauh M, Barrack M, Nichols J. Associations between the female athlete triad and injury among high school runners. Int J Sports Phys Ther 2014;9(7):948–58. Available at: https://www.ncbi.nlm.nih.gov/pmc/articles/PMC4275199. Accessed July 15, 2016.
7. Stickler L, Hoogenboom B, Smith L. The female athlete triad: what every physical therapist should know. Int J Sports Phys Ther 2015;10(4):563–71. Available at: https://www.ncbi.nlm.nih.gov/pubmed/26380148. Accessed July 15, 2016.
8. Thralls K, Nichols J, Barrack M, et al. Body mass-related predictors of the female athlete triad among adolescent athletes. Int J Sport Nutr Exerc Metab 2016;26(1): 17–25. Available at: https://www.ncbi.nlm.nih.gov/pubmed/26252427. Accessed July 15, 2016.
9. Laframboise M, Borody C, Stern P. The female athlete triad: a case series and narrative overview. J Can Chiropr Assoc 2013;57(4):316–26. Available at: https://www.ncbi.nlm.nih.gov/pmc/articles/PMC3845471. Accessed July 15, 2016.
10. Nazem TG, Ackerman KE. The female athlete triad. Sports Health 2012;4(4): 302–11. Available at: https://www.ncbi.nlm.nih.gov/pmc/articles/PMC3435916. Accessed July 15, 2016.

11. Gibbs JC, Williams NI, De Souza MJ. Prevalence of individual and combined components of the female athlete triad. Med Sci Sports Exerc 2013;45(5): 985–96. Available at: https://www.ncbi.nlm.nih.gov/pubmed/23247706. Accessed July 15, 2016.

12. Nichols JF, Rauh MJ, Lawson MJ, et al. Prevalence of the female athlete triad syndrome among high school athletes. Arch Pediatr Adolesc Med 2006;160(2): 137–42. Available at: https://www.ncbi.nlm.nih.gov/pubmed/16461868. Accessed July 15, 2016.

13. Reed JL, De Souza MJ, Williams NI. Changes in energy availability across the season in division I female soccer players. J Sports Sci 2013;31:314–24. Available at: https://www.ncbi.nlm.nih.gov/pubmed/23075047. Accessed July 15, 2016.

14. Cano Sokoloff N, Eguiguren M, Misra M, et al. Bone parameters in relation to attitudes and feelings associated with disordered eating in oligo-amenorrheic athletes, eumenorrheic athletes, and nonathletes. Int J Eat Disord 2015;48(5): 522–6. Available at: https://www.ncbi.nlm.nih.gov/pubmed/23075047. Accessed July 15, 2016.

15. Reed J, De Souza M, Kindler J, et al. Nutritional practices associated with low energy availability in division I female soccer players. J Sports Sci 2014;32(16): 1499–509. Available at: https://www.ncbi.nlm.nih.gov/pubmed/24787233. Accessed July 15, 2016.

16. Kroshus E, Sherman R, Thompson R, et al. Gender differences in high school coaches' knowledge, attitudes, and communication about the female athlete triad. Eat Disord 2014;22(3):193–208. Available at: https://www.ncbi.nlm.nih.gov/pubmed/24456303. Accessed July 15, 2016.

Sexuality Counseling for Women's Health Providers

Aleece Fosnight, MSPAS, PA-C, CSC, CSE

KEYWORDS

- Sexual health • Sexuality • Counseling • Education • Sexual function
- Sexual dysfunction • Women's health • Physician assistant

KEY POINTS

- Physician assistants play an important role in sexual medicine and sexuality counseling.
- There are 2 main models for sexuality counseling: PLISSIT (permission, limited information, specific suggestions, and intensive therapy) and DOUPE (description, onset, understanding, past, and expectations).
- An implementation of specific suggestions can enhance intimacy and sexuality.

INTRODUCTION

For many health care providers, the topic of sexual health was lacking during their education and training, despite a focus on gynecology and obstetrics, in which the vagina is a main focus of care. Patients are often surprised that the vagina is a main organ for sexual health and functioning. Secondary to shifts in culture and society, the topic of sexuality has become disconnected from medicine, with health care providers concerned that the topic of sexuality may feel like an invasion of their patients' privacy or may provoke sexual transference. However, in a 2009 national survey, 80% of women thought that sexual health was an important part of their overall health and 72% of women wanted to speak with their health care providers but often felt too embarrassed, with most of those women preferring that their health care providers bring up the topic of sexual health.[1,2] Physician assistants (PAs) are well suited to bring up and discuss sexual health and concerns with their patients, being able to spend more time on counseling during an office visit, understanding the biopsychosocial influences on sexual health functioning, as well as understanding the role of a sexual health team with referral sources to appropriate sexual health professionals when needed, including sex therapists and pelvic floor physical therapists.[1]

Disclosure: The author has no conflict of interest or financial disclosure.
Urology and Sexual Medicine, Pisgah Urology, Mission Medical Associates, 87 Medical Park Drive, Suite A, Brevard, NC 28712, USA
E-mail address: aleece.fosnight@gmail.com

Physician Assist Clin 3 (2018) 325–337
https://doi.org/10.1016/j.cpha.2018.02.002
2405-7991/18/© 2018 Elsevier Inc. All rights reserved.

physicianassistant.theclinics.com

BACKGROUND

With 43% of women in the United States having a sexual health concern,[2,3] health care providers are ill-equipped to meet the sexual health needs of their patients. When roughly 1 in 2 women walking through an office question their sexual functioning but do not feel comfortable bringing up the topic it becomes the provider's responsibility to help meet their need. There are several barriers to communication about sexual health on both the patient and provider sides. Patient barriers include shame, embarrassment, and fear of possible negative judgment by the provider, or assumption that the provider lacks the competence to discuss such issues.[4] However, 75% of patients want their providers to bring up their sexual health and feel more comfortable disclosing personal information because this normalizes the issue.[4] Provider barriers include embarrassment, lack of adequate time to address sexual concerns, insufficient training in sexual medicine to deal with their patients' concerns, and lack of treatment options for female sexual dysfunction.[4] Plus, providers may be dealing with their own sexual health concerns and feel uncomfortable discussing issues related to sexuality. In addition, sexuality carries its own set of cultural and societal taboos that have negative impacts on the way clinicians view sexual health and its importance to their patients.

DEFINITIONS

It might be thought that providers practicing in the specialty of obstetrics and gynecology would be proficient in discussing sexual health issues; however, most lack adequate education and training as well as struggling with understanding their own beliefs and values toward sexuality.[1] To better understand the relevance of discussing sexual health, it is essential to recognize that sexual health is a basic human right, established at birth.

The World Health Organization (WHO) defines sexual health as the "...state of physical, emotional, mental and social well-being in relation to sexuality. It is not merely the absence of disease, dysfunction or infirmity. Sexual health requires a positive and respectful approach to sexuality and sexual relationships, as well as the possibility of having pleasurable and safe sexual experiences, free of coercion, discrimination and violence. For sexual health to be attained and maintained, the sexual rights of all persons must be respected, protected, and fulfilled."

The American Sexual Health Association (ASHA) defines sexual health as the ability to embrace and enjoy sexuality throughout life. It is an important part of physical and emotional health. Being sexually healthy means:

- Understanding that sexuality is a natural part of life and involves more than sexual behavior.
- Recognizing and respecting the sexual rights that all people share.
- Having access to sexual health information, education, and care.
- Making an effort to prevent unintended pregnancies and sexually transmitted diseases and to seek care and treatment when needed.
- Being able to experience sexual pleasure, satisfaction, and intimacy when desired.
- Being able to communicate about sexual health with others, including sexual partners and health care providers.

THE BASICS

What is sexual health and what does it look like in a women's health setting? As seen through the definitions from the WHO and ASHA, sexual health is more than the absence of disease or unwanted pregnancy. Sexual health should also focus on body acceptance, consent, pleasure, and intimacy, all of which are basic human needs for survival and full satisfaction.[5] There are many changes throughout a woman's life cycle, including infant/toddler/child, prepubescent, puberty, reproductive, menses cycle, pregnancy, postpartum, lactation, perimenopause, menopause, and postmenopausal.[6] Sexual health functioning is multifactorial and can be affected by any or all of these changes. A thorough sexual history[5] (**Box 1**) is essential with each stage, can be implemented at any office visit, and should be part of the annual well-woman visit. The International Consultation in Sexual Medicine-5, a step-by-step algorithm, can also be helpful in evaluating and treating female patients with a sexual health concerns (**Fig. 1**).[7,8]

All health care providers should receive education and training in sexual health at the foundational level, including 3 specific components: desensitization and resensitization, knowledge building, and skill development.[6,9] The specific training is called a sexual attitude reassessment/restructuring (SAR) and helps health care providers overcome personal barriers to addressing sexual health in their practices. The SAR enables participants to assess their own beliefs, attitudes, and values toward sex and sexuality, which in turn facilitates comfort and ease of communication when discussing sexuality issues with patients.[9]

COUNSELING MODELS

One of the chief issues providers voice regarding sexual health concerns is the time constraint of this type of discussion.[4] However, there are many sexual health issues that are easy to assess and address through simple interventions without affecting patient flow. The Brief Sexual Symptom Checklist[7,8] (**Box 2**) is a simple triage tool that identifies patients who are interested in talking about their sexual health. This 6-item questionnaire can be incorporated into a patient intake form completed before the

---

Box 1
Sexual history

Taking a sexual history

- Are you currently involved in a sexual relationship?
- Do you have sex with men, women, both?
- Are you or your partner having any sexual difficulties at this time?

Additional questions

- Are you satisfied with your current sexual relationship?
- Do you have any sexual concerns you would like to discuss?

Follow-up questions

- Tell me about your sexual history: first sexual experiences, masturbation, number of partners, any sexually transmitted infections, any sexual problems, and any past sexual abuse or trauma.
- How often do you engage in sexual activity?
- What kinds of sexual activity do you engage in?

Data from Association of Reproductive Health Professionals. Talking to patients about sexuality and sexual health. What you need to know. 2008. Available at: http://www.arhp.org/Publications-and-Resources/Clinical-Fact-Sheets/Sexuality-and-Sexual-Health. Accessed December 5, 2017.

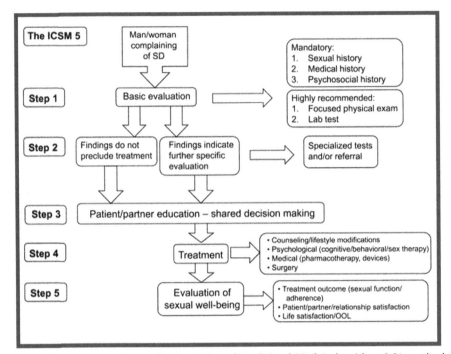

Fig. 1. The International Consultation in Sexual Medicine (ICSM)-5 algorithm. OOL, outlook on life; SD, sexual dysfunction. (*From* Hatzichrisou D, Rosen R, Derogatis LR, et al. Recommendations for the clinical evaluation of men and women with sexual dysfunction. J Sex Med 2010;7:346; with permission.)

appointment time. This questionnaire can lead the health care provider into 2 types of counseling models: PLISSIT (an acronym for the 4 levels of intervention: permission, limited information, specific suggestions, and intensive therapy[10]) and DOUPE (description, onset, understanding, past, and expectations).

Box 2
Brief sexual symptom checklist: women

Please answer the following questions about your overall sexual function:
1. Are you satisfied with your sexual function?
   ☐ Yes
   ☐ No. If no, please continue.
2. How long have you been dissatisfied with your sexual function? _____
3. The problems with your sexual function are: (mark all that apply)
   ☐ Problems with little or no interest in sex
   ☐ Problems with decreased genital sensation (feeling)
   ☐ Problems with decreased vaginal lubrication (dryness)
   ☐ Problems with reaching orgasm
   ☐ Problems with pain during sex
   ☐ Other: _____
4. Which problem (question 3) is most bothersome?
5. Would you like to talk about it with your health care provider?
   ☐ Yes
   ☐ No

From Hatzichrisou D, Rosen R, Derogatis LR, et al. Recommendations for the clinical evaluation of men and women with sexual dysfunction. J Sex Med 2010;7:346; with permission.

The PLISSIT model for sex therapy was developed by psychologist Jack Annon, and focuses on the idea that sexual health problems can be resolved with a basic 4-step process. The first 3 steps can be incorporated into a sexual health counseling session with the patient and then a referral can be made to a specialist, usually a sex therapist.

Permission

The first step gives patients permission to freely speak about their sexual health concerns. It also helps the provider validate the problem as a legitimate health concern, helping patients acknowledge that their feelings are justified and worthy of attention.[10] This step helps patients understand that sexual problems often result from negative emotions, such as anxiety, guilt, embarrassment, and self-consciousness. For example, a patient may be recently widowed and excited to be in a new relationship but continues to feel guilt and shame around engaging in intimacy with someone who is not her husband. The PA is perfectly suited to give the patient permission to feel conflicted about what to do but also able to give permission to move forward with her sexuality and experience sexuality with another human being. Applying this step in conversation with patients ensures that the patients establishes trust, allowing the patients to be honest with themselves, their partners, and their providers.

Limited Information

After permission giving, the provider is able to suggest LI on ways to improve the sexual health concern. This step is crucial in providing the patient with a small amount of information regarding the problem and/or question. The information may be anatomic, physiologic, or pathophysiologic to help provide background education for understanding, as well as to relieve anxiety or frustration.[10] For example, a patient may be concerned about dyspareunia and vaginal dryness. She may be 8 weeks post-partum and currently breastfeeding. Providing her with information regarding estrogen suppression from prolactin secondary to lactation causing her limited estrogen to her vaginal tissues, therefore leading to dryness of tissues, can help normalize her symptoms and validate her concern.

Specific Suggestions

The third step is crucial in pulling the pieces together and giving the patient answers to the sexual health concern. The provider is able to offer individualized tips, exercises, over-the-counter products, prescriptions, or recommendations used to treat the sexual health concern. This step is also vital to establish realistic expectations and goals for the patient, providing step-by-step instructions in moving forward to resolve the concern.[10] One of the most common reasons for sexual health concerns is lack of effective communication between partners.[11] With this third step, the provider is able to provide suggestions for patients to build their communication skills when discussing concerns with their partners. For example, a young, newly married woman with little sexual experience before her wedding night has difficulty achieving orgasm. One suggestion for her would be masturbation in order to find out key locations in the genital area that provide increased arousal and sensations. Once she is comfortable with self-exploration, the provider is able to help the patient move forward with communicating her needs and desires to her partner.

Intensive Therapy

For medical providers, this final step can be used in several different ways. It can be used by the provider, providing sexual health counseling through more advanced homework assignments and exercises, or could be a referral to other sexual health professionals.[7] These professionals include a sex therapist, especially when a psychological disorder is of concern, there has been an affair in the relationship, or there are unresolved issues around a past sexual assault or domestic abuse. Other referrals can include a pelvic floor physical therapist when there is hypertonicity in the pelvic floor muscles, birth trauma, pelvic pain, or the need for pelvic floor muscle strengthening. Health care professionals may also refer to other specialists such as a cardiologist, pulmonologist, neurologist, or endocrinologist for further work-up to evaluate sexual functioning when warranted.

Another model for sexual health counseling, the DOUPE model developed by Sallie Foley, LMSW, CST, allows professionals to gain information quickly and concisely, especially for integration of a sexual health assessment into a general office visit.[12]

Description

This is a quick assessment to isolate the patient's concern and surrounding situation. Simply asking the patient to describe the sexual health concern and circumstances around the concern helps to establish the foundation for the sexual health difficulty.

Onset

Understanding whether the sexual health difficulty has been lifelong or more recent allows the health care professional to explore reasons why the patient is having the problem. Also, is the issue paired with any other life event or change. For example, did the sexual health issue arise after a surgery or menopause, or after the birth of a child? It is also vital to recognize whether the sexual health concern occurs with every sexual encounter or with 1 person.

Understanding

Asking the patient to assess the concern helps the health care provider understand the level of distress and reasoning associated with the troubling situation. For example, the patient statement, "It's because God is punishing me," necessitates a different approach than if the patient said, "I believe this happens to men as they get older."[12]

Past

Asking questions about previous treatment options or ways the patient tried to fix the problem in the past can help the provider decipher new ways to approach treating the current sexual health concern and explore reasons why previous treatments did not improve the situation.[12] Most importantly, asking this question supports reasoning for why the patient is seeking help now.

Expectations

Assessing the patient's expectations for improvement helps to develop an action plan for treatment as well as setting realistic expectations in a time frame that fits the patient and provider goals.[12] Expectations can allow the health care provider to assess how motivated the patient is and what treatment obstacles may present themselves.

PATIENT POPULATIONS

Remember that sexual function and activity are shaped by a person's age, gender, availability of a partners, quality of the relationship, and overall health and lifestyle.[8] There are many patient populations that are seen as asexual or no longer sexually active; however, these are misconceptions.

Lesbian, Gay, Bisexual, Transgender, Queer/Questioning, Intersex, and Allies/Asexual

Over the past several years, lesbian, gay, bisexual, transgender, queer/questioning, intersex, and allies/asexual (LGBTQIA) health has gained heightened attention after the publication of the Healthy People 2020 goal, intended to decrease health disparities and promote quality care and health equity.[13,14] Although open discussion and recognition of personal biases are essential to all patient care, it is especially important to recognize and support a healthy self-concept of sexuality and sexual behaviors in this population, including the effects of cultural, institutional, and internalized stigma in providing appropriate health care to LGBTQIA patients. This goal can be difficult for some providers, and attending SAR training can help providers reflect on personal bias and how that affects their ability to take care of their patients.[9]

Many patients are not aware of the human immunodeficiency virus (HIV)/sexually transmitted infection (STI) risks associated with certain sexual behaviors. Education and counseling for prevention of HIV and STIs in LGBTQIA patients should focus on promoting healthy sexuality rather than disorders. Providers should have a plan to provide appropriate testing, vaccination, education, and counseling in a sex-positive environment that encourages sexual expression with emphasis on safer sex practices and harm reduction.[14]

Providers working with transgender patients should follow the *Standards of Care for the Health of Transsexual, Transgender, and Gender Noncomforming People, Version 7* (SOC), produced by the World Association for Transgender Health (WPATH).[13] The SOC also includes a section on sexual health and sexual functioning and should be readily available to clinicians. Transgender people face many significant barriers to adequate health care, including lack of health insurance, discrimination in the health care setting, and lack of competent medical providers, which can prevent sexual health discussions.[14] Although gender confirmation surgeries improve self-perception and body image, these surgeries do not necessarily extend to sexual functioning. Many patients encounter reduced arousal, inadequate lubrication, and pain during sexual activities.[14] Although postsurgical regret is low, it is important to discuss sexual functioning before surgery, during the transition process, and afterward.[13] When a provider is not competent to address these sexual health issues, it is still vital to raise the concern and refer to appropriate professionals who can help address the dysfunction. The SOC also recommends that transgender patients have a mental health professional to address psychological changes that occur during the transition process.[13]

Older Adults

Many health care providers believe that older adults are no longer sexual or that sexuality disappears after certain life events, causing barriers for this population when they seek assistance with sexual health concerns.[11] The National Survey of Sexual Health and Behavior study in 2010 at the Center for Sexual Health Promotion at the Indiana University School of Public Health found that most adults more than 65 years of age are engaging in many sexual activities and find sexual health very important to their overall health and well-being.[3] If older adults enjoyed sex in their early lives, it is reasonable that they will continue to enjoy sex later in life. Many older adults lacked sexual health education when they were younger, making up-to-date information addressing their concerns and treatment options critical. Assessment of sexual problems should be very similar to that of younger patients; however, there should be increased attention to comorbidities, medications, sleep, nutrition, exercise, memory, stress, isolation, partners, and social/family support.[12] Many older adults believe that there are no options for treatment of their sexual health concerns.[12] When discussing treatment options, first give permission to talk about sex and sexuality, establish comfort and trust, address specific concerns, teach distress tolerance and communication, and encourage a broader sense of success to include pleasure and satisfaction rather than function.[12]

Disabilities

There is a common misconception that people with disabilities do not engage in any type of sexual behavior. Disabilities can include physical, visual/auditory, mental, and intellectual, and patients with disabilities have a range of sexual desires and needs for sexual expression.[15] Those with physical disabilities have a range of sexual functionality and giving them permission to explore their range of sexuality through sex position modification, use of external vibratory and/or sexual enhancement devices, or even props can establish a sense of normalcy for the patient. Physical disabilities can include, but are not limited to, spinal cord injuries, arthritis, amputations, and multiple sclerosis. Many providers do not classify visual or auditory loss as a disability; however, these disabilities can be associated with significant lost function and many patients avoid sexual intimacy for fear of not being able to hear or see their partners.[15] It is important to recognize these disabilities as possible hurdles to sexual activity. For those patients with mental disabilities, including schizophrenia, bipolar, anxiety, substance abuse, and eating disorders, being vulnerable and open with a partner about their sexuality can be difficult. Many are self-conscious and avoid intimacy and relationships. Focus on self-awareness of sexuality and sexual functioning first before aiding the patient in becoming sexual with a partner, remembering that many medications for these disorders cause sexual dysfunction as well. Intellectual disabilities include autism, Asperger, Down syndrome, and fetal alcohol spectrum disorder. Although it can be difficult to determine whether those with intellectual disabilities have the capacity to decide to engage in sexual activity and/or give consent, sexual health is still a basic human right for all. It is important to discuss the potential for sexual activity with the patient's caregivers and guardians and help to find the best level of sexuality for the patient, ranging from self-stimulation to consensual coitus.[15] Discussions around pregnancy prevention, safe sex practices, and sexual assault should not be avoided.

SPECIFIC SUGGESTIONS

When looking for specific suggestions to provide the patient, it is important to be knowledgeable about various management strategies. Treatment plan options generally require the cooperation and participation of the patient's partner, which may focus on strengthening interpersonal communication and helping to discover and implement new ways to focus on the sexuality and intimacy of both partners.

Sensate Focus

One of the oldest forms of intimacy exercises, the sensate focus is among the mainstream treatments to aid couples refocus their thoughts to sensations and touch. Developed by Masters and Johnson in the late 1960s as a way for couples to reconnect to the sensory roots of sexuality, the sensate focus is a series of structured touching and exploratory exercises that provide opportunities for experiencing people's own personal and their partner's bodies in a nondemand fashion.[16] The exercises take couples through establishing mindfulness and purpose within their relationships and incorporate a step-by-step instruction focus on both receiving and giving touch.[16] Applying the sensate focus exercise into an office visit could be challenging; however, isolating specific patients who need to slow down their relationships and/or need to start back at the basics of their sexuality are perfect situations in which to prescribe this assignment. The provider may experience push-back from the couple with the amount of time that is needed; however, reassure them of the benefit and that reestablishing intimacy is about the journey not the destination.[16]

Role Play

Often, patients have a difficult time communicating and opening up to their partners or they may find it difficult to initiate the conversation about intimacy. Being able to role play communication techniques with patients can alleviate anxiety and build self-confidence for the patients.[6] Have the patient play their partner, because this brings out concerns that the patient thinks the partner would bring up, and the provider serves as the patient.

Kissing

Asking the patient about acts of kissing can clue the provider in on the interaction of touch between the patient and partner. Many couples that have been together longer than 1 year have forgotten the benefits of a long, passionate kiss. Often, secondary to busy schedules and familiarity, kissing becomes a peck on the lips or cheek. There are sensitive nerve endings in the lips that become heightened during kissing, prompting the limbic system (the pleasure-reward part of the brain) to release endorphins and dopamine: feel-good neurotransmitters in the brain.[11] It takes time to stimulate those nerves and it is suggested that a 1- minute to 2-minute kiss daily is needed to release those neurotransmitters.[11] Dopamine can also help to increase testosterone levels in the body, thereby increasing libido. There need to be limits to the kissing exercise. The thought of kissing may provoke anxiety in a patient who is concerned that the kiss will lead to more. There needs to be strict rules about not moving past kissing and to see this as foreplay for future intimate interactions. The kissing exercise can be applied to most patient encounters in which the connection between the patient and the partner has been lost; however, it is vital that the partner is aware that this is an exercise with limits and the provider needs to ensure cooperation from the partner.

Scheduling Intimacy

Work, family, and social obligations often leave little time for intimacy; however, this is no excuse. If the patient can schedule a coffee date with a friend, the patient can schedule a date night with the partner. Often, patients rebel against this exercise because they want their intimacy to be spontaneous, but, when reminded that they may have scheduled date nights earlier in the relationship, the thought of spontaneous intimacy becomes less of an issue. Although intimacy and/or sexual activity may or may not happen during the scheduled date night, the patient is simply holding space for the opportunity. There should not be any pressure for sexual activity to happen. Suggestions for a scheduling calendar include a daily 10-minute conversation about each other, 1 to 2 date nights a month, and at least 2 to 3 overnight dates a year; however, each intimacy schedule is individual and should ultimately be determined by the patient and/or couple.

Hand-Over-Hand Technique

When body image is a concern of the patient, or communication regarding what the patient would like to happen involving touch during intimacy, the hand-over-hand exercise can be helpful.[11] The patient uses a guiding technique with the partner's hand over the patient's, guiding them over areas of the body where they enjoy being touched. Then, hands are switched, and the partner's hand is on the bottom and the patient's hand over the top, again guiding to specific body areas of pleasure. This exercise can be particularly helpful for women who have undergone mastectomy for breast cancer or hysterectomy with or without bilateral salpingo-oophorectomy. This exercise can be combined with body mapping, in which the patient labels areas on the body where they enjoy being touched and areas that are off limits.

Journaling

When a patient presents with a sexual health concern but is struggling to voice apprehensions or communicate the concern with a partner, it can be easier for the patient to write the feelings and fears down. Once written, it may be easier to read concerns aloud to the partner in order to voice the relationship or sexuality worry. Journaling can also be extremely helpful in voicing wants, desires, and fantasies. Suggestions include having a desire jar in which strips of paper with sentences of desires are folded up and placed with scheduled times to act out the desire.

Self-stimulation

Secondary to most female reproductive organs being internal and the sociocultural views of being a "good girl," women are less likely to self-stimulate, or masturbate, versus their male counterparts, and often feel ashamed afterward, struggling with the pleasure it brought and fear of repeating the act. Not just body awareness but genital awareness is key for women to achieve sexual pleasure. Asking patients to reflect on what types of sexual activity and intimacy give them pleasure can help steer the patients into self-appreciation, which in turn allows them to voice their pleasure areas to their partners. Self-stimulation can incorporate digital stimulation, the use of an external vibratory device, and/or dilator. Self-stimulation also helps to promote optimal vulvovaginal health when integrating lubrication, moisturizer, and introitus stretching, as developed by Sallie Foley, LMSW, CST.[11] For women with vaginal atrophy and/or pelvic pain disorder, this approach can be very beneficial, especially for those who have never explored their genitals or their bodies.

Intimacy Without Intercourse

There are several medical conditions that do not allow intercourse; for example, vaginal atrophy, pelvic pain, and erectile dysfunction. With cues in the media, Hollywood, music, and magazines that focus on intercourse as being the ultimate goal, those unable to have penetrative sexual activity may feel abnormal, dysfunctional, and avoid intimacy altogether. Brainstorming alternatives to intercourse can give hope to patients. There are many ways that humans experience sexuality and intimacy, and intercourse is merely one of them. Discussing this with your patients can alleviate any anxiety or worry about not performing. This activity can also widen the patient's sexual repertoire.

Good-Enough Sex

Developed by Metz and McCarthy[17] in 2007, this model focuses on intimacy as the main goal, with pleasure as important as function and mutual emotional acceptance as the environment. Sex is integrated into daily life and daily life is integrated into sex life in order for the couple to develop their own unique sexuality. This model helps the couple to understand the ebbs and flows of sexuality. Establishing realistic expectations allows the couple to focus on the relationship rather than the sex. This focus can be accomplished at the office level by redirecting the couple to look at their overall relationship and not just 1 part of it.

> **Box 3**
> **Sexual health counseling guidelines**
>
> - Promote sexual health in clinical practice environments.
> - Provide patients with current information regarding sexual health.
> - Acknowledge patient's feelings, attitudes, and norms that may be obstacles to individual sexual health and use this information to help patients establish realistic goals.
> - Assist patients with development of skills they may need to achieve personal goals for sexual health: communication, negotiation, and planning strategies.
> - Participate in continuing education activities or trainings that focus on sexual health.
> - Be aware and respectful of patient's sexual values, beliefs, and lifestyles.
> - Understand how the values of health care providers or clinical staff/settings may influence practices in order to provide unbiased and comprehensive care.
>
> *Data from* Lamont J; Contributing authors. Female sexual health consensus clinical guidelines. J Obstet Gynaecol Can 2012;34(8):769–75; with permission.

Leave Out the Technology

Nowadays, it is rare to see someone without a cell phone. With the accessibility of technology literally at our fingertips, being attached to a device can sabotage even the healthiest of relationships. When there was a concern that partners were blatantly dependent on their devices, they were less satisfied with their relationships, stating that there was jealously over the cell phones with regard to the relationships their partners were having with their phones, and not with them.[18] Advise patients to put down the cell phone, tablet, or laptop, and pick up their partner's hand and have a conversation. In particular, leave the technology out of the bedroom. Although intimacy can happen anywhere, a couple's bedroom should be a sacred and safe space to embrace other another, not bask in the glow from a cell phone screen.

Although there are a myriad of other sexual health counseling tools and exercises for patients, those mentioned earlier are a good foundation for most patients and couples encountered by PAs in a women's health specialty. It is also beneficial to have a list of suggested books, Web sites, educational materials, and exercises in the examination room for quick accessibility, and these can be given to the patients for a seamless approach to counseling and building on the moment of communication. Although there are many tools available to women's health PAs for sexual health counseling, there are times when appropriate referrals need to be made. A sex therapist referral is appropriate for patients and/or couples dealing with a history of sexual assault/trauma, infidelity, affairs, out-of-control sexual behavior, or other psychological impacts on their sexuality.[7] Pelvic floor physical therapy is also a vital referral if pelvic pain, vaginismus, birth trauma, postsurgical event, or other anatomy-altering events have occurred. It is a good idea to have a list of the best clinicians available in your area and develop a good rapport with these providers, because they will refer to the provider as well in order to evaluate organic causes of sexuality difficulties. This approach is the basis for a sexual health team.

SUMMARY

In conclusion, it is evident that sexual health discussions are lacking in the women's health specialty clinic office setting. Women's sexual health has been deficient, and it is time to validate the importance of female sexuality and intimacy. PAs are well equipped to bring up the conversation; evaluate patients for sexual dysfunction; and provide high-quality, appropriate treatment of female patients. Sexual health is part of people's overall well-being and function. Addressing sexual health concerns and implementing a triage protocol can help alleviate patient and provider barriers. Focusing on the multifactorial influences that disrupt normal sexual functioning and building a sexual health team approach is the most effective way to support patients with concerns about their sexuality and intimacy. The sexual health counseling guidelines (**Box 3**)[6] can make talking about sex easier through practice and application of skills to promote honest and open communication to ensure the best possible care.

REFERENCES

1. Seaborne L, Prince R, Kushner D. Sexual health education in U.S. physician assistant programs. J Sex Med 2015;12(5):1158–64.
2. Swartzendruber A, Zenilman JM. A national strategy to improve sexual health. J Am Med Assoc 2010;304(9):1005–6.
3. Herbenick D, Reece M, Schick V, et al. Sexual behavior in the United States: results from a national probability sample of men and women ages 14-94. J Sex Med 2010;7:255–65.
4. Brandenburg U, Bitzer J. The challenge of talking about sex: the importance of patient-physician interaction. Maturitas 2009;63(2):124–7.
5. Association of Reproductive Health Professionals. Talking to patients about sexuality and sexual health. What you need to know. Sexual Health Fundamentals 2008.
6. Society of Obstetricians and Gynecologist of Canada. Female sexual health consensus clinical guidelines. J Obstet Gynaecol can 2012. No. 279.
7. Reisman Y, Porst H, Lowenstein L, et al. The ESSM manual of sexual medicine. 2nd edition. Amsterdam: Medix; 2015.
8. Hatzichrisou D, Rosen R, Derogatis LR, et al. Recommendations for the clinical evaluation of men and women with sexual dysfunction. J Sex Med 2010;7:346.
9. Britton P, Dunlap R. Designing and leading a successful SAR: a guide for sex therapists, sexuality educators, and sexologists. New York: Routledge; 2017.
10. Gee A, Gonzalez-Rivas S, Deshields T. Approaching the "Sex Talk": using Anon's PLISSIT model to address sexuality with a breast cancer patient. Pscyho-Oncology 2015;24:323.
11. Foley S, Kope S, Sugrue D. Sex matters for women: a complete guide to taking care of your sexual self. 2nd edition. New York: The Guilford Press; 2012.
12. Foley S. Biopsychosocial assessment and treatment of sexual problems in older age. Curr Sex Health Rep 2015;7:80–8.
13. Ettner R, Monstrey S, Coleman E. Principles of transgender medicine and surgery. New York: Routledge; 2016.
14. Makadon H, Mayer K, Potter J, et al. The Fenway guide to lesbian, gay, bisexual, and transgender health. 2nd edition. Philadelphia: American College of Physicians; 2015.
15. Eisenberg N, Andreski SR, Mona L. Sexuality and physical disability: a disability-affirmative approach to assessment and intervention within health care. Curr Sex Health Rep 2015;7(1):19–29.

16. Weiner L, Avery-Clark C. Sensate focus in sex therapy: the illustrated manual. New York: Routledge; 2017.
17. Metz M, McCarthy B. The "Good-Enough Sex" model for couple sexual satisfaction. Sex Relation Ther 2007;22(3):351–62.
18. Lapierre M, Lewis M. Should it stay or should it go now? Smartphones and relational health. Psychol Pop Media Cult 2016. https://doi.org/10.1037/ppm0000119.

Barriers to Use of Long-Acting Reversible Contraceptives in Adolescents

Meredith Browne, MMS, PA-C[a],*, Stevi Barrett, MMS, PA-C[b],
Laura Icenhour, MMS, PA-C[c], Suzanne Reich, PA-C, MPAS[d],
Rebecca Gimpert, MMS, PA-C[e], Tiffany Esinhart, MMS, PA-C[c]

KEYWORDS

- LARC • Contraception • IUD • Implant • Adolescence

KEY POINTS

- The American College of Obstetricians and Gynecologists and American Academy of Pediatrics endorse long-acting reversible contraceptives (LARCs) as the first-line contraceptive option for adolescents because of these agents' efficacy and safety profiles.
- Provider-based barriers to using LARCs include unfamiliarity with current guidelines, lack of training in insertion techniques, and misconceptions about the risks of infection and infertility.
- Providing patients with the opportunity for same-day intrauterine device (IUD) insertion increases their access to LARCs. Pregnancy must be ruled out before insertion.
- If IUD insertional pain is a concern, providers may offer a smaller framed IUD and/or a lidocaine paracervical block.

INTRODUCTION

In 2013 there were 448,000 annual pregnancies (43.4 per 1000 adolescents) in women 15 to 19 years old.[1] Despite this rate having decreased greatly over the past half century, the United States continues to have the highest rate of teen pregnancy among industrialized countries[2] (eg, **Fig. 1**). Most adolescent pregnancies are unintended.[2]

Disclosure: None of the authors have any financial or commercial affiliations to disclose.
[a] Obstetrics and Gynecology, Wake Forest Baptist Medical Center, Winston-Salem, NC 27157, USA; [b] Gastroenterology, Digestive Health Specialists, Winston-Salem, NC 27103, USA; [c] Emergency Medicine, US Acute Care Solutions, Carolinas Healthcare System, Charlotte, NC 28210, USA; [d] Department of PA Studies, Wake Forest School of Medicine, Medical Center Boulevard, Winston-Salem, NC 27157, USA; [e] Hospital Medicine, Carolinas Hospitalist Group, Carolinas Healthcare System, Charlotte, NC 28203, USA
* Corresponding author.
E-mail address: MeredithHBrowne@gmail.com

Physician Assist Clin 3 (2018) 339–352
https://doi.org/10.1016/j.cpha.2018.02.003
2405-7991/18/© 2018 Elsevier Inc. All rights reserved.
physicianassistant.theclinics.com

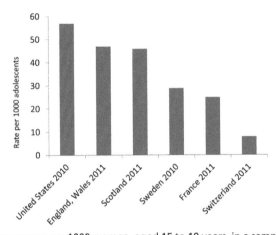

Fig. 1. Rates of pregnancy per 1000 women, aged 15 to 19 years, in a sampling of developed countries.

Given that the United States has a high teen pregnancy rate and that most teen pregnancies are unintended, there is justifiable consternation regarding low rates of effective contraception use in adolescents in the United States.

The American College of Obstetricians and Gynecologists (ACOG) and American Academy of Pediatrics (AAP) both endorse long-acting reversible contraceptives (LARCs) as the first-line option when counseling adolescents about contraception[3,4] because of these agents' high efficacy in preventing pregnancy, superior continuation rates, and limited contraindications.[3] Their recommendations state that providers should first introduce LARCs before other forms of contraception, including oral contraceptive pills (OCPs), transdermal patch, vaginal ring, and the depot medroxy-progesterone acetate (DMPA) injection.[3,4] Even with these organizations' recommendations, LARCs continue to be underused in the adolescent population, with only 5.8% of the female adolescents who use contraception reporting the use of LARCs.[5,6]

LARCs include the levonorgestrel-releasing intrauterine device (LNG-IUD), the copper intrauterine device (CuT380A), and the etonogestrel single rod implant (eg, **Table 1**). They are the most effective forms of contraception, with pregnancy rates of less than 1% per year, similar to that of permanent sterilization.[4] An important distinction between sterilization and LARCs is that any LARC can be removed at the discretion of the patient; this makes LARCs an ideal contraceptive choice for adolescents who would like to delay pregnancy for an extended period of time, but not permanently.

Adolescents, who have high rates of contraceptive failure, particularly need highly effective and low-maintenance contraceptive options.[7] Based on the 2011 to 2015 National Survey of Family Growth, 42.43% of female teenagers and 44.2% of male teenagers have participated in vaginal intercourse at least once in their lives.[6] In addition, adolescents report using less reliable forms of contraception: the most common being the male condom (97.4%) followed by coitus interruptus (69.7%), and then OCPs (55.5%).[6] The male condom has a failure rate as high as 18% and coitus interruptus as high as 22%.[3]

Even when adolescents use more reliable forms of birth control such as OCPs, they often do not use them properly.[3] Within the first year of OCP initiation, 5% to 9% of all users become pregnant, and this failure rate is nearly doubled in women younger than

Table 1
Food and Drug Administration–approved long-acting reversible contraceptives

LARC Type	Brand Name	Details	Duration	Contraindication
Etonogestrel implant	Nexplanon	68 mg. 35–45 μg/daily first year and decreases after 4 cm × 2 mm diameter rod	3 y	• Thromboembolic disorder • Liver disease • Progestin-sensitive cancer
Copper IUD (CuT380A)	Paragard	Nonhormonal 32 × 36 mm T frame	10 y	• Anatomic uterine abnormality • Active genital tract infection or within 3 mo of endometritis • Wilson disease • Uterine or cervical malignancy
LNG-IUD	Mirena	52 mg. 20 μg/daily 32 × 32 mm size	5 y	• Anatomic uterine abnormality • Gynecologic or breast cancer • Active genital tract infection or within 3 mo of endometritis • Liver disease
	Liletta	52 mg. 18.6 μg/daily 32 × 32 mm size	4 y	
	Skyla	13.5 mg. 14 μg/daily 28 × 30 mm size	3 y	
	Kyleena	19.5 mg. 17.5 μg/daily 28 × 30 mm size	5 y	

Abbreviation: IUD, intrauterine device.

21 years.[7,8] In contrast, LARCs have a low failure rate in all ages because they do not depend on user compliance.

An additional benefit to LARCs in adolescents is their high continuation rate compared with other contraceptives. In a study of women aged 14 to 45 years, the average 1-year continuation rate for LARCs was 85% with 80% user satisfaction.[9] When these results were stratified by age, there was no change in continuation rates for the LNG-IUD and implant with women less than 20 years old.[9] In contrast, 1 year continuation rates were 55.2% for OCPs, 56.5% for DMPA, 49.1% for the patch, and 54.2% for the ring.[9]

PERCEPTIONS ABOUT LONG-ACTING REVERSIBLE CONTRACEPTIVES
Patient Perceptions

A survey of young women aged 13 to 19 years showed their low overall knowledge about LARCs.[10] Of those studied, 53.9% had heard of the implant, 59.8% the LNG-IUD, and 46.1% the CuT380A.[10] Half of those surveyed did not know LARCs were the most efficacious contraceptives and thought incorrectly that LARCs negatively affect fertility.[10]

Adolescents gain most of their knowledge about contraception from personal anecdotes[11,12]; they are informed about a particular contraceptive based on acquaintances' experiences, whether positive or negative.[11,12] A qualitative survey revealed that adolescents recalled negative contraceptive experiences from friends and family more so than positive experiences.[13] This finding is significant because adolescents may be given incorrect or exaggerated information from peers that could affect their impression of LARCs.

However, in an additional qualitative study, many adolescents did report that information given to them by providers could potentially counteract acquaintances' anecdotes.[14] One study found that, if women were introduced to the IUD from a health care provider, they were 2.7 times more likely to choose them,[15] which suggests that, even if adolescents are first gaining information on contraception from peers, they still have a tendency to trust health care providers' recommendations. If providers are able to educate adolescents with correct and up-to-date information, adolescents may subsequently relay this accurate information to their peers.

Provider Perceptions

Medical providers who provide contraception for adolescents are typically those who practice in the specialties of pediatrics, family medicine, and obstetrics-gynecology. Pediatric providers account for most adolescent primary care, placing them in a unique position to be the first to introduce LARCs to this age group.[16] A survey of pediatricians regarding practices concerning LARCs showed a misunderstanding of the safety of IUDs in adolescents.[17] In a survey of 53 New York pediatricians, more than 80% reported initiating contraception, but only 35.8% reported counseling about IUD use.[18]

Lack of awareness of ACOG and AAP guidelines for LARC use in adolescents is not only evident for pediatric providers but also for obstetrician-gynecologists (OBGYNs). A survey of more than 1500 OBGYNs revealed that more than half disagreed with IUDs being the first-line choice of contraception for young women.[19] This survey also showed that OBGYNs who had recently completed continuing medical education or had read an ACOG publication were more likely to insert an IUD in a nulliparous woman.[19] Although this survey reveals that many OBGYNs are not up to date with current guidelines, it also suggests that education can help practitioners update their practices.[19]

One survey of family medicine residents found that most residents thought that an IUD was appropriate for a woman less than 20 years old, but only 51.8% of all residents thought that an IUD was appropriate for a woman who had contracted a sexually transmitted infection (STI) in the past 6 months, and nearly a third thought IUDs increase long-term risk of pelvic inflammatory disease.[20] Although the residents surveyed showed enthusiasm for IUDs, only 55.7% of first-year through third-year residents had inserted at least 1 LNG-IUD and only 31% had inserted at least 1 CuT380A.[20] In order for LARCs, and in particular IUDs, to be more available to adolescents, it is important to give resident physicians more opportunities to acquire the skills to perform insertions.

RISKS, BARRIERS, AND MISCONCEPTIONS OF LONG-ACTING REVERSIBLE CONTRACEPTIVES
Risk of Pelvic Inflammatory Disease with Intrauterine Devices

Pelvic inflammatory disease (PID) is an infection of the upper genital tract caused by the spread of bacteria (most commonly *Neisseria gonorrhoeae* and *Chlamydia trachomatis*) from the vagina or cervix to the uterus.[21] PID can lead to serious medical consequences such as tubo-ovarian abscess, ectopic pregnancy, and infertility.[21] The risk for PID is of concern for adolescents because this population has greater rates of STIs, which, if left untreated, predispose these patients to PID.[22] One study of OBGYNs showed that 1 in 7 of those surveyed thought that PID is a major risk of IUDs.[19] This association most likely stems from the chronicles surrounding the Dalkon Shield, an IUD that was shown in the 1970s to be associated with PID but has now been off the market for decades.[23]

There is also concern among some providers that insertion of an IUD for an adolescent already at increased risk for STIs may further increase the risk for acquiring PID.[24] Evidence shows that the small risk for PID after insertion is mildly increased for the 20 days after insertion but then returns to baseline.[25] It is thought that the likely cause of infection is contamination during the insertion procedure, not the IUD itself.[4,24,25]

An analysis of 6 studies investigating the relationship between IUD insertion and PID found that those women who had a cervical infection at the time of IUD insertion had a 0% to 5% risk of PID and those without a cervical infection at insertion had a 0% to 2% risk.[24] Although there seems to be a minimally increased risk of acquiring PID with IUD insertion in patients with a concurrent infection, one study showed there was no significant difference of PID after IUD insertion in adolescents who were screened for an STI within 1 year before IUD insertion compared with those who were not screened.[26] In addition, patients who were screened on the day of insertion, including those less than 26 years old, had similar rates of PID to those who were previously screened.[26] Therefore, an extra appointment for STI screening before IUD insertion is not necessary and is likely to lead to increased costs for the patient.[26] Adolescents should be screened for STIs at the time of IUD insertion.[27] They should be counseled about the small risk for infection and, in the case of infection, the patient can be safely treated with the IUD in place.[27]

Infertility

Another reservation about IUD use in adolescents is the fear that an IUD could lead to infertility.[12] Many adolescents are fearful the IUD will become permanently fixed in the body and unable to be removed.[12] A case control study of nulliparous women showed that CuT380A did not increase risk for tubal occlusion but that infection with C trachomatis did increase this risk.[23] An additional prospective study showed a quick return to fertility after IUD removal.[28] Providers should help dispel patients' fears that IUDs negatively affect future plans for pregnancy.

Expulsion of Intrauterine Devices

Historically, IUDs were marketed for parous women and this legacy may be a barrier to use in adolescents, who are likely to be nulliparous. OBGYNs are less likely to provide IUDs to nulliparous women.[19] Avoiding IUDs in nulliparous women may also be rooted in fear of difficulty of IUD placement and increased expulsion rates. In addition, young women express fear that an IUD expulsion would leave them susceptible to pregnancy.[12]

A study of IUD insertions in young women showed high success rates (>90%) for the insertion process.[29] In addition, the CHOICE study investigated IUD expulsions in thousands of women and found no increased expulsion rate in nulliparous women.[30] The study, however, did find an increased rate of expulsion in women less than 20 years of age, regardless of parity.[30] Although the rate was increased in this age group, their expulsion rate was low, at less than 3%.[30]

Expulsion of IUDs is highest for immediately postpartum women (within 10 minutes of placental delivery).[27] Despite this higher rate, ACOG recommends IUD and implant insertion in postpartum women before leaving the hospital.[27] Immediate insertion of LARCs is promoted given that postpartum women are motivated to begin contraception and may not return for their postpartum visits.[2]

Regardless of parity, young women should be counseled by their providers on the signs of an IUD expulsion and to do a monthly self-check of IUD placement to monitor themselves for expulsion.

Menstrual Cycle Disturbance with Long-Acting Reversible Contraceptives

Menstrual cycle disturbance is a common reason women decide to have their LARCs removed.[31] Each LARC method has a unique bleeding profile. Bleeding can be unpredictable for implant users and this change is the most common reason adolescents discontinue the implant.[4] Around 22% of women with the implant experience amenorrhea, 33% infrequent bleeding, 6.7% frequent bleeding, and 17.7% prolonged bleeding.[27]

Dysmenorrhea and heavy bleeding often increase in the first few months after CuT380A insertion but usually decrease over time.[27] In addition, irregular and increased bleeding is common in the first 3 months following insertion of LNG-IUDs but also usually decreases over time and may lead to amenorrhea.[27] LNG-IUDs with higher doses of levonorgestrel usually result in less bleeding over time.[27] The Mirena LNG-20 IUD is US Food and Drug Administration (FDA) approved to treat heavy menstrual bleeding and results in a 70% to 95% reduction in menstrual bleeding.[27] The use of nonsteroidal antiinflammatory medications is shown to improve dysmenorrhea and irregular/prolonged bleeding with all LARC methods.[27]

The CHOICE project surveyed women who experienced changes in menstrual flow and frequency of menses regarding their satisfaction with their contraception. At 6 months postinsertion, more than 90% of LARC users (95% of LNG-IUD users, 93% of CuT380A IUD users, and 90% of implant users) were satisfied with their form of birth control regardless of changes in bleeding.[32] Between 45% and 62% of LARC users report lighter bleeding and infrequent menses, which can be considered a benefit to LARC use.[32] Young women should be counseled regarding the unique bleeding changes associated with their chosen LARC.

Long-Acting Reversible Contraceptives Discontinuation

When compared with older women, adolescents have been found to have a slightly higher discontinuation rate of LARCs.[31] Although adolescents are slightly more likely to discontinue a LARC method, the rate of discontinuation is significantly lower than that of adolescents discontinuing non-LARC contraceptives.[31–33] An analysis of more than 10 studies showed a continuation rate of 84% for all LARC methods in adolescents.[34] Proper counseling about potential menstrual disturbances and coping mechanisms may reduce the discontinuation rate.[34] Specifically with the implant, adolescents should be counseled to promptly return to the office to discuss bleeding concerns, because this earlier consultation may improve continuation rates.[35]

Uterine Perforation with Intrauterine Device Insertion

Adolescents express concern that IUDs may cause harm to their bodies.[12] Uterine perforation is a potential adverse event, but it is uncommon.[36] A review of the safety of IUDs found that perforation rates of LNG-IUD and CuT380A were both very low, ranging from 0% to 0.1%, irrespective of age.[36] Women at the highest risk for perforation are those who are breast feeding and those who are postpartum (<36 weeks from last delivery).[37] Breastfeeding and postpartum state are independently associated with higher rates of IUD perforation.[37]

Although uterine perforation is a serious adverse event of IUD insertion, the outcomes of perforations in one study of more than 60,000 women were neither serious nor life threatening.[37] Providers should counsel their patients on the low risk for uterine perforation.

Fear and Pain of Intrauterine Device Insertion

Adolescents who have heard of the IUD, but who have not had an IUD themselves, express a fear of the insertion process.[12] Furthermore, adolescents fear not being in control during the procedure.[12] From the providers' perspective, some express concern that, if a young woman's first contraceptive is one that induces pain, she may be left with a negative impression of contraception and pelvic examinations.[38]

In order to reduce pain and increase ease of insertion, some providers administer misoprostol to nulliparous patients before IUD insertion.[39] A randomized study of adolescent nulliparous patients showed no reduction in pain or ease of insertion with prophylactic misoprostol.[39] The women pretreated with misoprostol experienced more adverse side effects like cramping and nausea before IUD insertion.[39] Routinely giving patients misoprostol before IUD insertion could worsen the IUD insertion experience and should be avoided.

Some providers require patients to be menstruating at the time of IUD insertion in order to definitively rule out pregnancy and because of the belief that insertion at this time may reduce pain and increase ease of the procedure.[40] A review of 8 studies showed no reduction of pain with IUD insertion while the patient was menstruating.[40] Because of the difficulty of scheduling appointments and arranging transportation, requiring a young woman to return while on her menses adds an unnecessary barrier to IUD use.

A 2017 randomized trial investigated the use of 10-mL 1% lidocaine paracervical nerve blocks in reducing pain of the 13-mg LNG-IUD (Skyla) in young women.[41] Those women who received a paracervical block rather than a sham block reported less pain with insertion.[41] In addition, a comparison of LNG-IUDs found that the models of LNG-IUD that contain a smaller frame caused less pain with insertion and were easier to insert in younger women.[42]

To reduce pain during IUD insertion, providers may offer a smaller IUD, such as Kyleena19.5-mg LNG-IUD or Skyla 13.5-mg LNG-IUD, as well as administration of a paracervical block.[41,42] IUDs may be safely and effectively inserted at any point in the menstrual cycle as long as pregnancy can be excluded.[40] In order for an adolescent to feel in control of the insertion process, providers should reassure the patient that she may request discontinuation at any point during the procedure.

Cost of Long-Acting Reversible Contraceptives

Patients who are uninsured or whose insurance plans do not cover LARCs may be deterred from pursuing these methods. In one study, when the cost of LARCs was eliminated, 67% of women chose one of these as their method of contraception.[43] Providers also express concern about the cost of LARCs, specifically citing low reimbursement from private and public insurers.[38] Although the up-front cost of LARCs can be high, the long-term savings of choosing LARCs are significant, not only for individuals but also for the US health systems as a whole.[44]

For clinics whose concern is low reimbursement for LARCs from insurers, there is a newer LNG-IUD that was designed specifically to reduce this barrier.[45] The Liletta 52-mg LNG-IUD is available for $50 for practices eligible for 340B pricing. For practices not eligible for these benefits, the price of this LNG-IUD is still lower than for other LNG-IUDs.[45]

With the current Patient Protection and Affordable Care Act's (ACA) emphasis on preventive health, LARCs are covered by most insurance plans.[46] Women who are uninsured, however, must pay high out-of-pocket costs for an LARC.[44] For these women, practices can offer payment plans or can refer patients to publicly funded clinics.[4] In addition, patients can be made aware of the ARCH (Access and Resources in Contraceptive Health) patient assistance program.[47] This program provides Bayer LNG-IUDs at no charge to women who are uninsured or whose plans do not cover IUDs and who meet certain financial criteria.[47]

SOLUTIONS TO BARRIERS AND MISCONCEPTIONS

Although there are many barriers to LARC use in adolescents, one solution is to increase provider and patient education. To help decrease teen pregnancy rates, providers should stay up to date on evidence-based guidelines regarding LARC use in adolescents. Providers educated on LARC guidelines for adolescents change their behaviors.[19] When counseling adolescents on contraceptive options, providers should discuss LARCS first, before other less effective contraceptives (eg, **Fig. 2**).[3,4] Providers should be educated on appropriate candidates for IUDs including adolescents, nulliparous women, and those with a history of STIs and PID (eg, **Table 2**).[4]

There is evidence that patient education increases the use of LARCs.[19] Although adolescents are heavily influenced by the contraceptive experience of their peers, they

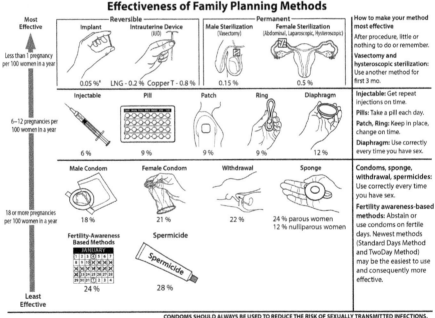

Fig. 2. Efficacy of contraceptives with typical use. [a] The percentages indicate the numbers out of every 100 women who experienced an unintended pregnancy within the first year of typical use of each contraceptive method. (*Adapted from* World Health Organization (WHO) Department of Reproductive Health and Research, Johns Hopkins Bloomberg School of Public Health/Center for Communication Programs (CCP). Knowledge for Health project. Family planning: a global handbook for providers (2011 update). Baltimore (MD): CCP and WHO; 2011; and Trussell J. Contraceptive failure in the United States. Contraception 2011;83:397–404; and Available at: https://www.cdc.gov/reproductivehealth/contraception/unintendedpregnancy/pdf/Contraceptive_methods_508.pdf.)

Table 2
Intrauterine device misconceptions and recommendations

Misconceptions	Recommendations
PID	• There is a small risk for PID (<5%) after IUD insertion[24] • Screen for STIs on the day of insertion; testing before IUD insertion is unnecessary[26] • Same-day insertion of IUDs is safe if there is no sign of cervicitis[26] • In the case of infection, patient may be treated without removing IUD[27]
Infertility	• There is a quick return to fertility after IUD removal[28]
Expulsion	• Expulsion of IUD in nulliparous adolescents is low (<3%)[30]
Insertion	• Insertion of IUDs in nulliparous adolescents is highly successful (>90%)[29] • LARCs may be inserted at any time in menstrual cycle as long as pregnancy is excluded
Perforation	• Risk of uterine perforation with IUD insertion is low (<0.1%)[36]
Pain	• Misoprostol and insertion of IUD on menses does not decrease pain or increase ease of insertion[39,40] • Lidocaine paracervical block and smaller framed IUDs decrease pain of IUD insertion[41,42]

Data from Refs.[24,26–29,36,39–42]

do trust advice given to them by their medical providers.[11,12,14] If providers inform their young patients about the benefits and potential side effects of LARCs, these women in turn can teach their peers. These chains of communication may help increase the overall acceptance of LARCs.

LARCs should be an accessible form of contraception for adolescents. To improve accessibility, providers who treat adolescent patients, particularly pediatric providers, should be trained on insertion of LARCs so that patients need not be referred elsewhere for these services. In addition, when pregnancy can be excluded, same-day insertion should be offered.

The two most common reasons for IUD discontinuation in young women are bleeding changes and pain.[48] Young women who are interested in LARCs should be counseled on possible bleeding changes and encouraged to return when problems arise, because this improves continuation rates.[35]

Young women who are uninsured, whose insurance plans do not cover IUDs, or who are concerned about confidentiality when using their parent's insurance should be encouraged to go to publicly funded health clinics or apply to the ARCH assistance program.[4,47] Practices with concerns for high costs/low reimbursement for LARCs may consider ordering the Liletta LNG-IUD, because this is the least expensive IUD option available.[45]

A 2017 study investigated the use of a tablet app with women aged 12 to 18 years and its effect on their intention to use effective contraception.[49] The study used the app Health-E-You, which contained interactive materials focusing on the individual's need for contraception, as well as resources to teach adolescents about the recommendations for contraception[49] The study showed that app users had an increased interest in LARC methods.[49] Because the Internet is such a prevalent part of teen culture, this app promises to be an effective avenue to educate young women.

Some providers express concern related to clinic time constraints reducing their ability to thoroughly counsel their patients.[38] Providers may improve adolescent knowledge of LARC methods and use less clinic time if they implement app-based programs as well as providing printed brochures.[38,49]

SUMMARY

Adolescents continue to use less effective methods such as condoms, withdrawal, and OCPs for contraception despite the recommendation by ACOG and AAP for preferential use of LARCs for adolescents. Data show that LARCs are the most cost-effective contraceptives available in the United States, despite their higher up-front costs.[44] LARCs are safe and effective contraception options for young women. Providers can be reassured that misconceptions about IUDs, such as increased risk of PID, difficulty of placement in nulliparous patients, association with infertility, and likelihood of uterine perforation with insertion, have been dispelled in multiple studies[36]

In order to effectively implement LARC use in their practices, providers must be trained on appropriate counseling as well as the insertion and removal process of these methods. The training of pediatric providers should be especially encouraged because they deliver proportionally more of the medical care to adolescents, while concomitantly feeling the least comfortable with contraceptive counseling.[16,18] In order to maintain trust between the provider and patient and to improve continuation rates, providers should counsel patients about LARC insertion procedures as well as any potential side effects. Providers should remind patients of the high efficacy and long-term use of LARCs, and together they should discuss options for decreasing pain during IUD insertion.[48]

Although this article seeks to highlight barriers to LARCS, it is important to highlight patient concerns about provider bias regarding LARCs.[50] Women express concern that providers undervalue their individual perspectives and do not respect their concerns about side effects or their decisions about removing LARCs.[50] Providers must be cognizant of the history of reproductive abuses in marginalized women and empathetically respond to women who develop LARC side effects.[4,50]

Provider education regarding the benefits, risks, and limited contraindications of LARCs is essential in reducing teen pregnancy. Once educated, providers may confidently counsel patients in accordance with AAP and ACOG guidelines and become better advocates for their young patients' health.

REFERENCES

1. Kost K, Maddow-Zimet I, Arpaia A. Pregnancies, births and abortions among adolescents and young women in the United States, 2013: national and state trends by age, race and ethnicity. Guttmacher Institute. New York: Guttmacher Institute; 2017. Available at: https://www.guttmacher.org/report/us-adolescent-pregnancy-trends-2013.
2. Sedgh G, Finer LB, Bankole A, et al. Adolescent pregnancy, birth and abortion rates across countries: levels and recent trends. J Adolesc Health 2015;5(2): 223–30. Available at: https://www.ncbi.nlm.nih.gov/pubmed/?term=1.%09Sedgh +G%2C+Finer+LB%2C+Bankole+A%2C+Eilers+MA%2C+Singh+S.+Adoles cent+Pregnancy%2C+Birth+and+Abortion+Rates+Across+Countries%3A.
3. Braverman P, Adelman W, Alderman E, et al. Contraception for adolescents. Pediatrics 2014;134(4):e1244–56. Available at: http://pediatrics.aappublications. org/content/pediatrics/134/4/e1244.full.pdf.
4. American College of Obstetrics and Gynecologists. Committee opinion no. 539: adolescents and long-acting reversible contraception: implants and intrauterine devices. Obstet Gynecol 2012;1(10):983–8. Available at: https://www.acog.org/ ~/media/Committee%20Opinions/Committee%20on%20Adolescent%20Health %20Care/co539.pdf.

5. Branum AM, Jones J. Trends in long-acting reversible contraception use among U.S. women aged 15–44. NCHS Data Brief 2015;(188):1–8. Available at: https://www.ncbi.nlm.nih.gov/pubmed/25714042.

6. Abma JC, Martinez GM. Sexual activity and contraception use among teenagers in the United States, 2011-2015. Natl Health Stat Report 2017;104:1–23. Available at: https://www.cdc.gov/nchs/data/nhsr/nhsr104.pdf.

7. Winner B, Peipert JF, Zhao Q, et al. Effectiveness of long-acting reversible contraception. N Engl J Med 2012;366(21):1998–2007. Available at: https://www.ncbi.nlm.nih.gov/pubmed/22621627.

8. Kost K, Singh S, Vaughan B, et al. Estimates of contraceptive failure from the 2002 National Survey of Family Growth. Contraception 2008;77(1):10–21. Available at: https://www.ncbi.nlm.nih.gov/pmc/articles/PMC2811396/.

9. Peipert JF, Zhao Q, Allsworth JE, et al. Continuation and satisfaction of reversible contraception. Obstet Gynecol 2011;117(5):1105–13. Available at: https://www.ncbi.nlm.nih.gov/pubmed/21508749.

10. Hoopes AJ, Ahrens KR, Gilmore K, et al. Knowledge and acceptability of long-acting reversible contraception among adolescent women receiving school-based primary care services. J Prim Care Community Health 2016;7(3):165–70. Available at: https://www.ncbi.nlm.nih.gov/pubmed/27067583.

11. Greenberg KB, Jenks SC, Piazza N, et al. A snapshot of urban adolescent women's contraceptive knowledge at the onset of a community long-acting reversible contraceptive promotion initiative. J Pediatr Adolesc Gynecol 2017; 30(4):474–8. Available at: https://www.ncbi.nlm.nih.gov/pubmed/28088438.

12. Potter J, Rubin SE, Sherman P. Fear of intrauterine contraception among adolescents in New York City. Contraception 2014;89(5):446–50. Available at: https://www.ncbi.nlm.nih.gov/pubmed/?term=potter+fear+of+intrauterine+contraception.

13. Anderson N, Steinauer J, Valente T, et al. Women's social communication about IUDs: a qualitative analysis. Perspect Sex Reprod Health 2014;46(3):141–8. Available at: https://www.ncbi.nlm.nih.gov/pmc/articles/PMC4245018/.

14. Hoopes AJ, Gilmore K, Cady J, et al. A qualitative study of factors that influence contraceptive choice among adolescent school-based health center patients. J Pediatr Adolesc Gynecol 2016;29(3):259–64. Available at: https://www.ncbi.nlm.nih.gov/pubmed/26477942.

15. Fleming KL, Sokoloff A, Raine TR. Attitudes and beliefs about the intrauterine device among teenagers and women. Contraception 2010;82(2):178–82. Available at: https://www.ncbi.nlm.nih.gov/pubmed/20654760.

16. Freed GL, Dunham KM, Gebremariam A, et al. Which pediatricians are providing care to America's children? An update on the trends and changes during the past 26 Years. J Pediatr 2010;157(1):148–52.e1. Available at: https://www.ncbi.nlm.nih.gov/pubmed/20227714.

17. Berlan ED, Pritt NM, Norris AH. Pediatricians' attitudes and beliefs about long-acting reversible contraceptives influence counseling. J Pediatr Adolesc Gynecol 2017;30(1):47–52. Available at: https://www.ncbi.nlm.nih.gov/pubmed/27639750.

18. Rubin SE, Cohen HW, Santelli JS, et al. Counseling adolescents about the intrauterine contraceptive device: a comparison of primary care pediatricians with family physicians and obstetrician-gynecologists in the Bronx, New York. J Prim Care Community Health 2015;6(3):162–9. Available at: https://www.ncbi.nlm.nih.gov/pubmed/25628297.

19. Luchowski AT, Anderson BL, Power ML, et al. Obstetrician–gynecologists and contraception: practice and opinions about the use of IUDs in nulliparous women,

adolescents and other patient populations. Contraception 2014;89(6):572–7. Available at: https://www.ncbi.nlm.nih.gov/pubmed/24679477.

20. Schubert FD, Herbitter C, Fletcher J, et al. IUD knowledge and experience among family medicine residents. Fam Med 2015;47(6):474–7. Available at: https://www.ncbi.nlm.nih.gov/pubmed/26039766.

21. Centers for Disease Control and Prevention. Pelvic inflammatory disease: CDC fact sheet. Available at: https://www.cdc.gov/std/pid/stdfact-pid.htm. Accessed October 15, 2017.

22. Datta SD, Torrone E, Kruszon-Moran D, et al. Chlamydia trachomatis trends in the United States among persons 14 to 39 years of age, 1999-2008. Sex Transm Dis 2012;39(2):92–6. Available at: https://www.ncbi.nlm.nih.gov/pubmed/22249296.

23. Hubacher D, Lara-Ricalde R, Taylor DJ, et al. Use of copper intrauterine devices and the risk of tubal infertility among nulligravid women. N Engl J Med 2001; 345(8):561–7. Available at: https://www.ncbi.nlm.nih.gov/pubmed/11529209.

24. Mohllajee AP, Curtis KM, Peterson HB. Does insertion and use of an intrauterine device increase the risk of pelvic inflammatory disease among women with sexually transmitted infection? A systematic review. Contraception 2006;73(2):145–53. Available at: https://www.ncbi.nlm.nih.gov/pubmed/16413845.

25. Farley TM, Rosenberg MJ, Rowe PJ, et al. Intrauterine devices and pelvic inflammatory disease: an international perspective. Lancet 1992;339(8796):785–8. Available at: http://www.ncbi.nlm.nih.gov/pubmed/1347812.

26. Sufrin CB, Postlethwaite D, Armstrong MA, et al. *Neisseria gonorrhea* and *Chlamydia trachomatis* screening at intrauterine device insertion and pelvic inflammatory disease. Obstet Gynecol 2012;120(6):1314–21. Available at: http://www.ncbi.nlm.nih.gov/pubmed/23168755.

27. American College of Obstetricians and Gynecologists. Long acting reversible contraception: implants and intrauterine devices. Practice bulletin no. 186. Obstet Gynecol 2017;130(5):e251–69. Available at: https://www.acog.org/Resources-And-Publications/Practice-Bulletins/Committee-on-Practice-Bulletins-Gynecology/Long-Acting-Reversible-Contraception-Implants-and-Intrauterine-Devices.

28. Hov GG, Skjeldestad FE, Hilstad T. Use of IUD and subsequent fertility: follow-up after participation in a randomized clinical trial. Contraception 2007;75(2):88–92. Available at: https://www.ncbi.nlm.nih.gov/pubmed/17241835.

29. Bayer LL, Jensen JT, Li H, et al. Adolescent experience with intrauterine device insertion and use: a retrospective cohort study. Contraception 2012;86(5): 443–51. Available at: https://www.ncbi.nlm.nih.gov/pubmed/22560185.

30. Madden T, McNicholas C, Zhao Q, et al. Association of age and parity with intrauterine device expulsion. Obstet Gynecol 2014;124(4):718–26. Available at: https://www.ncbi.nlm.nih.gov/pubmed/25198262.

31. Modesto W, Bahamondes MV, Bahamondes L. A randomized clinical trial of the effect of intensive versus non-intensive counselling on discontinuation rates due to bleeding disturbances of three long-acting reversible contraceptives. Hum Reprod 2014;29(7):1393–9. Available at: https://www.ncbi.nlm.nih.gov/pubmed/24812309.

32. Diedrich JT, Desai S, Zhao Q, et al. Association of short-term bleeding and cramping patterns with long-acting reversible contraceptive method satisfaction. Am J Obstet Gynecol 2015;212(1):50.e1-8. Available at: https://www.ncbi.nlm.nih.gov/pmc/articles/PMC4275360/.

33. Rosenstock JR, Peipert JF, Madden T, et al. Continuation of reversible contraception in teenagers and young women. Obstet Gynecol 2012;120(6):1298–305. Available at: https://www.ncbi.nlm.nih.gov/pubmed/23168753.

34. Diedrich JT, Klein DA, Peipert JF. Long-acting reversible contraception in adolescents: a systemic review and meta-analysis. Am J Obstet Gynecol 2017;216(4): 364.e1–12. Available at: https://www.ncbi.nlm.nih.gov/pubmed/28038902.

35. Dickson J, Hoggart L, Newton VL. Unanticipated bleeding with the etonogestrel implant: advice and therapeutic interventions. J Fam Plann Reprod Health Care 2014;40(3):158–60. Available at: https://pdfs.semanticscholar.org/8fe9/995c67ae8514300e0060519b02d3eff689aa.pdf.

36. Jatlaoui TC, Riley HE, Curtis KM. The safety of intrauterine devices among young women: a systematic review. Contraception 2017;95(1):17–39. Available at: https://www.ncbi.nlm.nih.gov/pubmed/27771475.

37. Heinemann K, Reed S, Moehner S, et al. Risk of uterine perforation with levonorgestrel-releasing and copper intrauterine devices in the European Active Surveillance Study on Intrauterine Devices. Contraception 2015;9(4):274–9. Available at: http://www.sciencedirect.com.go.libproxy.wakehealth.edu/science/article/pii/S0010782415000086.

38. Kavanaugh ML, Frohwirth L, Jerman J, et al. Long-acting reversible contraception for adolescents and young adults: patient and provider perspectives. J Pediatr Adolesc Gynecol 2013;26(2):86–95. Available at: https://www.ncbi.nlm.nih.gov/pmc/articles/PMC3672067/.

39. Edelman AB, Schaefer E, Olson A, et al. Effects of prophylactic misoprostol administration prior to intrauterine device insertion in nulliparous women. Contraception 2011;84(3):234–9. Available at: https://www.ncbi.nlm.nih.gov/pubmed/21843686.

40. Whiteman MK, Tyler CP, Folger SG, et al. When can a woman have an intrauterine device inserted? A systematic review. Contraception 2013;87(5):666–73. Available at: https://www.ncbi.nlm.nih.gov/pmc/articles/PMC4578632/.

41. Akers AY, Steinway C, Sonalkar S, et al. Reducing pain during intrauterine device insertion: a randomized controlled trial in adolescents and young women. Obstet Gynecol 2017;130(4):795–802. Available at: https://www.ncbi.nlm.nih.gov/pubmed/28885425.

42. Gemzell-Danielsson K, Schellschmid I, Apter D. A randomized, phase II study describing the efficacy, bleeding profile, and safety of two low-dose levonorgestrel-releasing intrauterine contraceptive systems and Mirena. Fertil Steril 2012; 97(3):616–22. Available at: https://www.ncbi.nlm.nih.gov/pubmed/22222193.

43. Secura GM, Allsworth JE, Madden T, et al. The contraceptive CHOICE project: reducing barriers to long-acting reversible contraception. Am J Obstet Gynecol 2010;203(2):115.e1-7. Available at: http://www.ncbi.nlm.nih.gov/pmc/articles/PMC2910826/.

44. Trussell J, Henry N, Hassan F, et al. Burden of unintended pregnancy in the United States: potential savings with increased use of long-acting reversible contraception. Contraception 2013;87(2):154–61. Available at: http://www.ncbi.nlm.nih.gov/pubmed/22959904.

45. Kattan DR, Burkman RT. Your teenage patient and contraception: think "long acting" first. OBG Manag 2015;27(9):22–4, 26–9. Available at: http://www.mdedge.com/obgmanagement/article/102325/contraception/your-teenage-patient-and-contraception-think-long-acting.

46. Birth control benefits. Healthcare.gov. Available at: https://www.healthcare.gov/coverage/birth-control-benefits/. Accessed October 15, 2017.

47. ARCH Patient Assistant Program. Available at: http://www.archpatientassistance.com/. Accessed October 15, 2017.

48. Friedman JO. Factors associated with contraceptive satisfaction in adolescent women using the IUD. J Pediatr Adolesc Gynecol 2015;28(1):38–42. Available at: https://www.ncbi.nlm.nih.gov/pubmed/25555299.

49. Mesheriakova VV, Tebb KP. Effect of an iPad-based intervention to improve sexual health knowledge and intentions for contraception use among adolescent females at school-based health centers. Clin Pediatr 2017;56(13):1227–34. Available at: https://www.ncbi.nlm.nih.gov/pubmed/28950721.

50. Higgins JA, Kramer RD, Ryder KM. Provider bias in long acting reversible contraception (LARC) promotion and removal: perceptions of young adult women. Am J Public Health 2016;106(11):1932–7. Available at: https://www.ncbi.nlm.nih.gov/pubmed/27631741.

Understanding Polycystic Ovarian Syndrome

Emily S. Edmondson, MPAS, PA-C*

KEYWORDS

- Polycystic ovarian syndrome • Ovarian cysts • Obesity • Insulin resistance
- Hyperandrogenism • Metabolic syndrome • Gestational diabetes

KEY POINTS

- Polycystic ovarian syndrome is a condition that crosses multiple specialties and, with a wide range of presentations, should be understood by the entire medical community.
- The cause and pathogenesis of polycystic ovarian syndrome are not entirely known and therefore require more evidence-based research to be better understood.
- Polycystic ovarian syndrome diagnosis and treatment are focused on the patient's symptoms, and there is no one treatment that is accepted as superior.
- Early diagnostic approach and symptomatic treatment by the patient's health care team can make it possible for appropriate management and a promising prognosis.

INTRODUCTION

Polycystic ovarian syndrome (PCOS) is a heterogeneous disease that affects many aspects of the patient's endocrine system, and the patient's reproductive, dermatologic, and psychological systems.[1] PCOS was first explained in 1935 when American gynecologists Dr Irving F. Stein, Sr. and Dr Michael L. Leventhal recounted seven female patients who presented with symptoms of hyperandrogenism and oligomenorrhea or amenorrhea. These patients also had bilateral polycystic ovaries. When these gynecologists performed a bilateral wedge resection on the patients' ovaries, there was a therapeutic effect: the patients' irregular menses and issues with fertility were normalized. Therefore, the two gynecologists concluded that the cause of the disease lay in the dysfunction of polycystic ovaries, hence the name "polycystic ovarian syndrome."[2]

PCOS is one of the most common metabolic disorders in premenopausal women.[3] It is estimated that the prevalence rate of this disease is 5% to 10%. However, there is also evidence that this rate is actually underestimated. This could be caused by

Disclosure Statement: The author has no conflicts of interest or disclosures to declare.
Vineyard Primary Care, UPMC Hamot, 2060 North Pearl Street, North East, PA 16428, USA
* 3952 Ridge Parkway, Erie, PA 16510.
E-mail address: edmondsone2@upmc.edu

Physician Assist Clin 3 (2018) 353–362
https://doi.org/10.1016/j.cpha.2018.02.004
2405-7991/18/© 2018 Elsevier Inc. All rights reserved.

physicianassistant.theclinics.com

providers underdiagnosing the disease.[1] Regardless, what must be pointed out and kept in mind when discussing this disease is the relevance it has today. According to the Centers for Disease Control and Prevention, the obesity rate in the United States is 34%. Although that statistic has been steady since 2007, it still includes a large number of American citizens. Combined with the prevalence of overweight individuals, that statistic jumps up to around 66% of Americans who are above their ideal weight. These statistics impact the discussion regarding PCOS because diseases associated with obesity and being overweight, such as type 2 diabetes mellitus (T2DM) and risk factors for cardiovascular disease, are also associated with PCOS.[4,5]

CAUSE AND PATHOGENESIS
Cause

The cause of PCOS is unknown. It is thought that there are many factors influencing the ultimate outcome of a female developing the disease. However, there is believed to be a strong genetic influence in the development of PCOS. Various animal models have shown evidence that fetal exposure to increased maternal androgen is associated with the development of PCOS later in life. Also, studies done on families of adolescent girls with PCOS found that their fathers had an obesity rate of 94% and a metabolic syndrome (MetS) rate of 79%. In that same study, the mothers of those patients had a 54.4% rate of being obese and a 34% rate of having MetS. This links the significance of today's obesity rates and the genetic influence on the development of PCOS.[2]

Another idea is that changes or exposures that occur during childhood and puberty may play a role in the development of the condition. The production of steroids by the ovaries is thought to play a role in the development of PCOS, specifically in infancy during periods of increased insulin-like growth factor 1 production. Hormonal changes during puberty are also thought to play a role in the cause of PCOS, either because of the increase in androgen production during puberty or simply atypical brain development. The latter is thought to result in atypical puberty and therefore abnormal hormonal production.[6]

Pathogenesis

There is no definite pathogenesis that has been uncovered in all patients with PCOS. As with the cause, there seems to be many genetic and environmental factors that cause the metabolic and reproductive changes associated with PCOS. However, one characteristic that many patients with PCOS possess is insulin resistance. Insulin resistance, and subsequent hyperinsulinemia, are prevalent in 50% to 70% of patients with PCOS. Hyperinsulinemia has a negative effect on regulation of lipid metabolism, protein synthesis, and modification of androgen production, resulting in some of the typical signs and symptoms associated with PCOS.[3]

Androgen production modification is a result of the dysregulation of luteinizing hormone. Luteinizing hormone is dysregulated at the central level when there is an increased amount of insulin in the bloodstream. This dysregulation occurs because increased insulin levels support an increase in the activity of cytochrome P-450 C17 in the liver, which results in an increase in androgen secretion by the ovaries.[7]

The modification of androgen production leads to androgen excess in the body. That androgen excess results in hypersensitivity of the androgen receptor gene that is located on the X chromosome. The androgen receptor gene codes for an androgen receptor protein that contains repeats of the nucleobases CAG. These CAG repeats are polymorphic and range from 8 to 35 repeats. It has been shown that the fewer number of CAG repeats, the more severe PCOS symptoms seem to be, so the CAG repeats and PCOS symptoms have an inverse relationship.[8]

Another contributing theory to the development of PCOS is that of the adipokine adiponectin, resulting in a protective effect on developing obesity. Some of the benefits adiponectin has on the body include insulin sensitizing, fat burning, antioxidant, and antiatherogenic properties. Compared with theca cells of normal ovaries, the theca cells of polycystic ovaries have a decreased number of adiponectin receptors, which can have an effect on increasing obesity and ultimately increasing androgen levels.[9] Again, the exact pathogenesis of PCOS is not identified and may include a variable combination of the theories discussed, lending to the difficulty of identifying a distinct causative pathway.

HISTORY AND PHYSICAL EXAMINATION
History

Patients who are ultimately diagnosed with PCOS usually present first with one, or a combination, of these three symptoms or chief complaints: (1) hirsutism, (2) weight gain, or (3) amenorrhea.[5] Of course, the patient could present to a primary care provider for any of these complaints. However, if complaining of hirsutism, the patient may present to a dermatology provider or an endocrinology provider; if complaining of weight gain, the patient may present to an endocrinology provider; if complaining of amenorrhea, the patient may present to a gynecology provider. This is important in relating the disease back to its heterogeneous characteristics and realizing that providers of many different specialties could have to examine, diagnose, treat, or refer a patient who is suffering from PCOS, highlighting the importance of universal knowledge of this condition across all specialities.[1] Additional signs and symptoms of PCOS are found in **Table 1**.

On further questioning, it is typically found that the patient's family history is positive for cardiovascular or endocrine diseases, such as T2DM, hypertension, or another coronary artery disease. It is also likely that the patient's family history is positive for PCOS because it is accepted as hereditary. Along with a family history, it is important to ask the patient questions about her past medical history, including endocrine or gynecologic disorders, and medications. These could cause symptoms similar to what is seen with PCOS; therefore, it is important to rule them out.[5]

Table 1	
Signs and symptoms of polycystic ovarian syndrome	
Signs	**Symptoms**
• Type 2 diabetes mellitus	• Acne
• Hypertension	• Seborrhea
• Insulin resistance	• Hirsutism
• Acanthosis migrans	• Irregular menses
• Nonalcoholic liver disease	• Infertility
• Obstructive sleep apnea	• Alopecia
• Imbalanced luteinizing hormone/follicle-stimulating hormone ratio	• Obesity

Signs and symptoms not specific to PCOS.
Data from Madnani N, Khan K, Chauhan P, et al. Polycystic ovarian syndrome. Indian J Dermatol Venereol Leprol 2013;79:310–21

Social history of dietary habits is also important to assess when interviewing a patient who might have PCOS. A study done in 2014 that compared the dietary habits of adolescent girls with a diagnosis of PCOS with those without a diagnosis of PCOS determined that the girls with PCOS had worse dietary habits. These conclusions came from the higher sugar intake and caloric intake by the girls with PCOS. These girls also had a higher tendency to eat more total fat, monounsaturated and polyunsaturated fats, and cholesterol. The girls with PCOS were found to eat more out of pleasure, which can possibly result in overeating and increased caloric intake.[10]

Physical Examination

If PCOS is suspected, physical examination of the patient includes a thorough skin examination to check for hirsutism, acne, alopecia, and pigmentation changes. The skin examination allows the provider to evaluate the endocrine system symptoms that may be present with PCOS. A pelvic examination should also be performed on every patient suspected to have PCOS. On the pelvic examination, the provider should palpate for any bilateral pelvic masses and inspect for clitoromegaly.[2] Positive findings indicate further work-up to possibly diagnose PCOS.

DIAGNOSIS

Although there have been many organizations with diagnostic criteria for PCOS, the most commonly used to diagnose PCOS is the Rotterdam criteria of 2003. The diagnostic criteria set forth by this body have three components: (1) oligo-ovulation and/or anovulation (oligomenorrhea or amenorrhea), (2) clinical and/or biochemical signs of hyperandrogenism, and (3) polycystic ovaries on ultrasound. There needs to be at least 12 ovarian cysts measuring 2 to 9 mm in size on each ovary to meet the criteria of polycystic ovaries.[2] On ultrasound, the polycystic ovaries present as the classic "string of pearls."[11] The patient must present with two of the three criteria to be diagnosed with PCOS.[2] Other diagnostic criteria used to diagnose PCOS, along with a summary of the Rotterdam criteria, are found in **Table 2**.

Besides the presence of multiple cysts on the ovaries, the other diagnostic criteria for PCOS are also similar in girls who are going through puberty. Therefore, attempting to make a diagnosis of PCOS in an adolescent girl is difficult. There are some recommendations for diagnosing PCOS in adolescent girls that ensure that the diagnosis of PCOS is appropriate rather than misinterpreted signs and symptoms of puberty.

Table 2
Diagnostic criteria for PCOS

National Institutes of Health (1990)	Rotterdam Criteria (2003)	Androgen Excess Society (2006)
Must include both • Oligo-ovulation or anovulation • Signs of hyperandrogenism (clinical or biochemical)	Must include 2 of 3 • Oligo-ovulation or anovulation • Signs of hyperandrogenism (clinical or biochemical) • Polycystic ovaries on ultrasound[a]	Must include • Oligo-ovulation or anovulation with or without polycystic ovaries on ultrasound • Signs of hyperandrogenism (clinical or biochemical)

[a] There need to be at least 12 ovarian cysts measuring 2 to 9 mm in each ovary.
Must exclude other causes of signs and symptoms.
Data from Madnani N, Khan K, Chauhan P, et al. Polycystic ovarian syndrome. Indian J Dermatol Venereol Leprol 2013;79:310–21.

Oligomenorrhea should be present for at least 2 years before considering the biochemical signs of hyperandrogenism as an accurate diagnostic criterion for PCOS. The adolescent girls who have these signs of hyperandrogenism should be monitored and re-evaluated once annually, because they are at an increased risk of PCOS. As with adults, obesity, insulin resistance, and hyperinsulinemia are not diagnostic criteria for PCOS in adolescent girls.[12]

Before one can officially make the diagnosis of PCOS, there are some differential diagnoses that need to be ruled out. These differentials are produced based on the presenting symptoms of the patient and include disorders of the reproductive and endocrine system. **Table 3** includes these differential diagnoses, the symptoms that are similar between these diagnoses and PCOS, and the diagnostic tests that are used to rule them out.[13]

TREATMENT
Lifestyle Modifications

Treatment of PCOS is complex; there is no single treatment method that results in discontinuation of symptoms and normalization of endocrine and reproductive imbalances for every patient. In addition, there is no definitive cure for this disease. Rather, the treatment approach is focused on treating the symptoms of the disease.[2] First-line treatment for PCOS is lifestyle modification, such as weight loss via dieting or exercising. It has been shown that even a 5% weight loss can improve PCOS symptoms, and a 1% decrease in body mass index (BMI) can improve insulin resistance.[2,14,15] Physical activity can also improve mental health in patients with PCOS by decreasing prevalence of depression and anxiety. The exact mechanism of this is unknown.[16,17]

Progressive resistance training is an exercise program that has been shown to positively affect insulin sensitivity in patients with PCOS. This training program works to improve skeletal muscle size and quality via metabolic capacity, which in turn improves insulin sensitivity. This is possible because skeletal muscle is the largest reservoir for insulin-stimulated glucose disposal. Patients could be advised to challenge their skeletal muscles by using free-weights or machine weights and using multiple resistance exercises that target several muscle groups. These can be repeated two to three times weekly, giving the muscles 48 to 72 hours of rest between sessions. It has been shown that in patients with obesity and T2DM, insulin sensitivity is

Table 3
Differential diagnoses for PCOS

Differential Diagnosis	Symptoms in Common	Laboratory Tests to Differentiate
• Pregnancy	• Amenorrhea	• hCG pregnancy test
• Prolactinoma	• Amenorrhea	• Prolactin
• Hypothyroidism	• Amenorrhea, weight gain	• TSH and free T4
• Cushing syndrome	• Hirsutism, obesity	• 24-h urine free cortisol
• Hyperthecosis	• Ovarian cysts on US	• Total testosterone
• Ovarian tumor	• Ovarian cysts on US	• Total testosterone
• Adrenal tumor	• Hyperandrogenism	• DHEA-S
• Late-onset CAH	• Hyperandrogenism	• 17-Hydroxyprogesterone

Abbreviations: CAH, Congenital Adrenal Hyperplasia; DHEA-S, Dehydroepiandrosterone-sulfate; hCG, human chorionic gonadotropin; TSH, thyroid-stimulating syndrome; US, ultrasound.
Data from Sheehan MT. Polycystic ovarian syndrome: diagnosis and management. J Clin Med Res 2004;2(1):13–27.

increased by more than 45% after 16 weeks of progressive resistance training.[18] Another form of exercise that has been shown to improve PCOS symptoms is holistic yoga. Twelve weeks of a holistic yoga program could decrease hormone levels that cause the negative effects of PCOS.[19]

Medications

If lifestyle modifications are not effective at reducing symptoms of PCOS, medication is also an option. Metformin is one choice for long-term maintenance of PCOS symptoms. Use of metformin results in decreased serum androgen and an improvement in ovulatory and menstrual frequency. Glucose intolerance can also be treated with metformin.[2,20] Another medication option in the management of PCOS symptoms is pioglitazone. A comparative study performed in India showed that pioglitazone is actually superior to metformin in restoring the menstrual cycle, improving ovulatory rate, decreasing the clinical signs of hyperandrogenism, and preventing or delaying T2DM.[7] Ultimately, the patient would notice more benefit from using metformin or pioglitazone along with lifestyle modifications if lifestyle modifications alone were not beneficial.[2]

Treatment of menstrual irregularity has also been achieved by using combination hormonal oral contraceptives, and possibly progesterone-only contraception methods. Treatment of anovulation has been achieved in up to 85% of patients, with rates of pregnancy being anywhere from 30% to 50% by using the ovulation induction medication clomifene (Clomid).[15] It is necessary to treat anovulation not only to improve conception rates but also because anovulation is associated with hyperandrogenism and unopposed estrogen, which can lead to endometrial hyperplasia, increasing the risk for endometrial cancer. The administration of hormonal contraceptive methods or depot medroxyprogesterone acetate (Provera) converts the endometrium from proliferative to secretory, protecting the patient from endometrial hyperplasia and ultimately decreasing the risk of endometrial cancer.[21]

Additional Treatment Options

Alternative and complementary medicine may be a treatment route that certain patients prefer, so it is wise for providers to understand the options available regarding this treatment method. Acupuncture is one such method that can be considered in patients who show no or limited benefit from lifestyle modification and medication. When compared with the side effects and adverse reactions that may result from medications, acupuncture is a safe treatment option. In a systematic study that spanned 30 years of clinical investigation, abdominal acupuncture was used to assess the abdominal points and their relation to the whole body. In this study, it was shown that the abdominal acupuncture directly affected adipose tissue and provided somatic innervation that directly corresponded to the uterus and ovaries. This is expected to restore normal endocrine and metabolic function of the ovaries. Also, compared with metformin, abdominal acupuncture was shown to improve menstrual frequency, BMI, and waist-to-hip ratio.[22]

COMPLICATIONS AND PROGNOSIS

A patient with PCOS is at a higher risk for many endocrine and reproductive complications, including T2DM, cardiovascular disease, hypertension, dyslipidemia, MetS, and endometrial cancer. Therefore, it is important to screen these patients regularly for signs and symptoms of these diseases.[2,3] There are no formal guidelines for screening patients with PCOS for these cardiometabolic complications; however, it is in the provider's and the patient's best interests to monitor certain parameters to avoid these complications.

Multiple physical and psychological complications can accompany a PCOS diagnosis. T2DM can develop if the insulin resistance is not well-controlled. Cardiovascular disease risk is increased because of modifications in the biosynthesis of steroids, cholesterol, and lipids. Breast and endometrial cancers can also result from PCOS. The increased risk of breast and endometrial cancers results from the hyperinsulinemia. Insulin works as a mitogenic, which can result in a proliferative effect. This can result in the presence of oncogenes and benign tissue being transformed into malignant tissue.[7,23]

Psychological complications of PCOS include depression, anxiety, poor self-esteem, eating disorders, and psychosexual dysfunctions.[24] It has been discovered that women with PCOS are at an increased risk of developing symptoms they describe as depression and anxiety, which can lead to major depressive disorder and general anxiety disorder, compared with women without PCOS. Although appropriate treatment of psychological complications associated with PCOS has not been determined, it is suspected that a cognitive behavioral therapy program might be beneficial for these patients. Because of the physical changes that present with PCOS, such as obesity, hirsutism, and acne, lifestyle modifications, such as diet modification, exercise, and coping strategies, can help to prevent suffering from depression and anxiety in these patients.[25]

During pregnancy, the risk of developing gestational diabetes mellitus and pregnancy-induced hypertension are increased in patients with PCOS.[7,26] Women with PCOS are two times as likely to develop gestational diabetes mellitus compared with women without PCOS. To decrease the development of gestational diabetes and the complications that accompany this condition, obstetric providers should recommend following a stricter diet and controlling excessive weight gain for patients with PCOS.[27]

Although the prevalence of PCOS in the female population is 5% to 10% of premenopausal women, that prevalence rate increases to 50% in women who are considered to be subfertile. These women typically require assistance in achieving pregnancy, including lifestyle changes, laparoscopic ovarian drilling, or ovulation induction via medications. In some cases, more complex intervention is required, such as controlled ovarian hyperstimulation or in vitro fertilization (IVF). Complications with controlled ovarian hyperstimulation, such as high cost of medications and risking ovarian hyperstimulation syndrome, may result in less favorable outcomes compared with IVF; however, this has yet to be confirmed. Women with PCOS who are unable to achieve success with IVF may benefit from in vitro maturation. In vitro maturation seems to be more favorable over IVF in women with PCOS compared with women without PCOS. Therefore, pregnancy is possible but more complicated in women with PCOS compared with women without PCOS.[28]

Screening Tools for Complications

BMI is one helpful screening tool that is used to predict complications associated with obesity, such as MetS, hirsutism, and acne. Blood pressure should be taken at each visit with every patient because of the increased risk of cardiovascular events when combined with obesity.[29] In fact, one known but uncommon complication associated with PCOS is idiopathic intracranial hypertension. The exact relationship has yet to be determined, but the rate of PCOS in women with idiopathic intracranial hypertension is five- to eight-fold greater than women who have PCOS in the general population.[30] Monitoring glucose metabolism via oral glucose tolerance test is important in these patients because 25% of adolescents with PCOS have irregularities in their glucose metabolism, independent of their BMI.[29]

Prognosis

If any of these psychic or psychological issues arise, it is important to treat them promptly to prevent further complications and to increase the chances for a favorable prognosis. If these comorbidities and complications are ignored, there is an increased chance for the patient to have a less than desirable prognosis. Otherwise, the prognosis for patients with PCOS is promising.[2,3]

SUMMARY

Despite the discovery of PCOS more than 80 years ago, there are still many unanswered questions regarding the cause, pathogenesis, diagnosis, and treatment of this condition. The heterogeneity and intricacy of this condition play a role in hypotheses that have flaws in all aspects. Although this does not take away from the validity of the existence of this condition, it does make it more difficult to diagnose and treat.[6] There are differential diagnoses that must be excluded to support a diagnosis of PCOS, and treatment is difficult to master because of the unknown cause and the need to treat the symptomatology rather than the disease as a whole.[2,13–15] Ultimately, more research studies are needed to better understand the origin of this condition and what can be done to effectively treat one of the most common metabolic disorders in reproductive-age women and its metabolic and cardiovascular effects.[6] Because of the connection PCOS has with obesity, it is important to recognize that the prevalence of this disease could be on the rise.[4] However, with prompt teamwork by the patient's primary care provider, endocrinology provider, gynecology provider, dermatology provider, and nutritionist, this disease is manageable and can offer the patient a positive prognosis.[1]

REFERENCES

1. Tomlinson J, Letherby G, Pinkney J, et al. Raising awareness of polycystic ovarian syndrome. Nurs Stand 2013;27(40):35–9.
2. Madnani N, Khan K, Chauhan P, et al. Polycystic ovarian syndrome. Indian J Dermatol Ve 2013;79(3):310–21.
3. Prasad Pothina N, Jennings P. The link between diabetes and polycystic ovary syndrome. Pract Nurs 2013;24(3):120–2.
4. Gagnon M, Stephens MB. Obesity and national defense: will America be too heavy to fight? Mil Med 2015;180(4):464–7.
5. Kulshreshtha B, Singh S, Arora A. Family background of diabetes mellitus, obesity, and hypertension affects the phenotype and first symptom of patients with PCOS. Gynecol Endocrinol 2013;29(12):1040–4.
6. Popescu I, Ionescu C, Dimitriu M, et al. Controversies in polycystic ovarian syndrome. Gineco.eu 2017;13(1):42–5.
7. Devi AS, Anuradha J. Metformin and pioglitazone in polycystic ovarian syndrome: a comparative study. IAIM 2017;4(7):39–44.
8. Rajender S, Carlus SJ, Bansal SK, et al. Androgen receptor CAG repeats length polymorphism and the risk of polycystic ovarian syndrome (PCOS). PLoS One 2013;8(10):1–12.
9. Comim FV, Hardy K, Franks S. Adiponectin and its receptors in the ovary: further evidence for a link between obesity and hyperandrogenism in polycystic ovarian syndrome. PLoS One 2013;8(11):1–9.

10. Eleftheriadou M, Stefanidis K, Lykeridou K, et al. Dietary habits in adolescent girls with polycystic ovarian syndrome. Gynecol Endocrinol 2015;31(4):269–71.

11. Catteau-Jonard S, Bancquart J, Poncelet E, et al. Polycystic ovaries at ultrasound: normal variant or silent polycystic ovary syndrome? Ultrasound Obstet Gynecol 2012;40(2):223–9.

12. Elnashar A. An evidence based approach for diagnosis of adolescent polycystic ovarian syndrome. Middle East Fertil Soc J 2016;21(3):194–5.

13. Sheehan MT. Polycystic ovarian syndrome: diagnosis and management. J Clin Med Res 2004;2(1):13–27.

14. Mahoney D. Lifestyle modification intervention among infertile overweight and obese women with polycystic ovary syndrome. J Am Assoc Nurse Pract 2014; 26(6):301–8.

15. Costello MF, Misso ML, Wong J, et al. The treatment of infertility in polycystic ovary syndrome: a brief update. Aust N Z J Obstet Gynaecol 2012;52(4):400–3.

16. Conte F, Banting L, Teede H, et al. Mental health and physical activity in women with polycystic ovary syndrome: a brief review. Sports Med 2015;45(4):497–504.

17. De Frene V, Verhofstadt L, Lammertyn J, et al. Quality of life and body mass index in overweight adult women with polycystic ovary syndrome during a lifestyle modification program. JOGNN 2015;44(5):587–99.

18. Cheema BS, Vizza L, Swaraj S. Progressive resistance training in polycystic ovary syndrome: can pumping iron improve clinical outcomes? Sports Med 2014;44(9): 1197–207.

19. Nidhi R, Padmalatha V, Nagarathna R, et al. Effects of a holistic yoga program on endocrine parameters in adolescents with polycystic ovarian syndrome: a randomized controlled trial. J Altern Complement Med 2013;19(2):153–60.

20. Hamed HO. Role of adiponectin and its receptor in prediction of reproductive outcome of metformin treatment in patients with polycystic ovarian syndrome. J Obstet Gynaecol Res 2013;39(12):1596–603.

21. Binette A, Howatt K, Waddington A, et al. Ten challenges in contraception. J Womens Health 2017;26(1):44–9.

22. Zheng YH, Wang XH, Lai MH, et al. Effectiveness of abdominal acupuncture for patients with obesity-type polycystic ovary syndrome: a randomized controlled trial. J Altern Complement Med 2013;19(9):740–5.

23. Salilew-Wondim D, Wang Q, Tesfaye D, et al. Polycystic ovarian syndrome is accompanied by repression of gene signatures associated with biosynthesis and metabolism of steroids, cholesterol and lipids. J Ovar Res 2015;8(1):1–14.

24. Shorakae S, Boyle J, Teede H. Polycystic ovary syndrome: a common hormonal condition with major metabolic sequelae that physicians should know about. Intern Med J 2014;44(8):720–6.

25. Correa J, Sperry S, Darkes J. A case report demonstrating the efficacy of a comprehensive cognitive-behavioral therapy approach for treating anxiety, depression, and problematic eating in polycystic ovarian syndrome. Arch Womens Ment Health 2015;18(4):649–54.

26. Wang Y, Zhao X, Zhao H, et al. Risks for gestational diabetes mellitus and pregnancy-induced hypertension are increased in polycystic ovary syndrome. Biomed Res Int 2013;2013:182582.

27. Pan M-L, Chen L-R, Tsao H-M, et al. Relationship between polycystic ovarian syndrome and subsequent gestational diabetes mellitus: a nationwide population-based study. PLoS One 2015;10(10):1–9.

28. Siristatidis C, Sergentanis TN, Vogiatzi P, et al. In vitro maturation in women with vs. without polycystic ovarian syndrome: a systematic review and meta-analysis. PLoS One 2015;10(8):1–19.

29. Davista A. PCOS in adolescents: beyond the reproductive implications. Contem OB/GYN 2013;58(12):63–6.

30. Shin SH, Kim YM, Kim HY, et al. Idiopathic intracranial hypertension associated with polycystic ovarian syndrome. Pediatr Int 2014;56(3):411–3.

Benign Breast Disease

Tiffany Riley, MPAS, PA-C*

KEYWORDS

- Benign breast disease • Fibroadenoma • Breast cyst • Breast pain

KEY POINTS

- Approximately 50% of women have benign breast disease at some point in their lifetime.
- Risk of breast cancer increases with some types of benign breast disease.
- Diagnostic imaging varies based on clinical evaluation and age of patient.

INTRODUCTION

Approximately 50% of women have some type of benign breast disease (BBD) over the course of their lifetime.[1] With the increased emphasis on screening mammograms, the frequency of biopsies showing BBD has also risen. Although most nonproliferative benign breast lesions do not pose future risk for breast cancer, proliferative lesions without atypia and proliferative lesions with atypia do increase risk for future breast carcinoma. This risk increases substantially for women with a strong family history of breast cancer. This article reviews breast anatomy and diagnostic imaging techniques, and discusses the various types of BBD including cause, risk factors, management, and future risk of breast carcinoma.

BREAST ANATOMY AND DEVELOPMENT

The mature adult breast lies between the second and sixth ribs above the pectoralis muscle. Breast tissue also extends into the axilla as the tail of Spence. The breast is composed of skin; subcutaneous tissue; and mammillary tissue, which consists of epithelial and stromal components.[2,3]

The breast is made of 12 to 20 lobes, and each lobe is made of 20 to 40 smaller lobules. The lobules are in turn made of 10 to 100 milk-producing acini that drain into terminal ducts. These merge into small lactiferous ducts attached to each lobule, which branch together to form larger ducts. These larger ducts carry milk toward the nipple. Each of the major ducts widens to form an ampulla deep to the nipple, then narrows to form an individual opening in the nipple (**Fig. 1**). The ducts comprise the epithelial components of the breast. Most benign and malignant breast diseases originate in the acini and terminal duct structures.

670 W Shepard Lane, Farmington, UT 84025, USA
* 2027 Ribbon Lane, Salt Lake City, UT 84117.
E-mail address: tiffpriley@yahoo.com

Physician Assist Clin 3 (2018) 363–371
https://doi.org/10.1016/j.cpha.2018.02.005
2405-7991/18/© 2018 Elsevier Inc. All rights reserved.

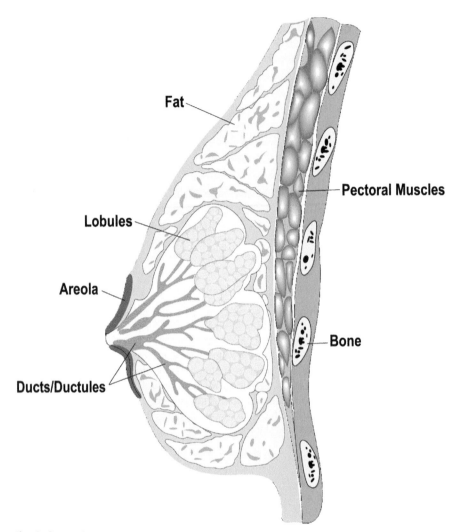

Fig. 1. Breast Anatomy.

The functional glandular tissue is surrounded by the breast stroma, which consists of adipose and fibrous connective tissue. Fibrous bands called Cooper ligaments connect the superficial and deep pectoral fascia surrounding the breast and are a natural support for the breast.

The skin of the breast contains hair follicles, sebaceous glands, and exocrine sweat glands. The areola is a circular pigmented zone measuring 15 to 60 mm in diameter. Morgagni tubercles are located on the areola, and are the openings to the ducts of the Montgomery glands, which are large sebaceous glands that provide lubrication for the nipple. The nipple has abundant nerve endings and smooth muscle tissue, which surrounds the lactiferous ducts.

The main blood supply of the breast stems from the internal mammary artery and the lateral thoracic arteries. Lymphatic drainage is superficial and deep, and flows toward the axillary, internal mammary, and clavicular lymph nodes.

Primitive ductal elements are present at birth, and begin to undergo changes during puberty. Terminal ends of the primitive ducts enlarge and develop alveolar buds and ductules, which form the lobules. Changing levels of estrogen and progesterone during the menstrual cycle stimulate the evolution of more mature lobules. This process takes many years and the breasts are not fully mature until a full-term pregnancy occurs.

Breast tissue also undergoes periodic changes throughout the menstrual cycle. During the premenstrual phase, increased estrogen and progesterone levels cause the acinar epithelial cells to increase in number and size. The ductal lumens widen, causing slight increase in breast size and breast tenderness in many women. This is followed by menstruation and the postmenstrual phase in which the breast acini decrease in number and size, and the lactiferous ducts also shrink in diameter.

EVALUATION OF A BREAST MASS

Breast masses may be discovered by the patient on self-breast examination, by the medical provider on clinical breast examination, or noted on screening mammogram. Women presenting with a breast mass should have a detailed history taken, including clinical history of the mass, evidence of nipple discharge or skin changes, associated tenderness or trauma, medications, relationship to the menstrual cycle, and family history of breast disease. A thorough breast examination with inspection and palpation of the breast must be completed, noting the size, shape, consistency, mobility, and location of the mass.

Diagnostic imaging of breast masses depends on clinical suspicion and age of the patient. Women older than age 40 should be evaluated initially with diagnostic mammography and supplemented with breast ultrasound as indicated. Women younger than age 30 tend to have very dense breast tissue, limiting the usefulness of mammography. For young women, ultrasound is the preferred method of initial breast imaging. MRI is another method of breast imaging, and has extremely high sensitivity for detection of cancer. MRI is reserved for high-risk patients and those with suspected malignancy.

Mammogram and ultrasound findings are reported by the Breast Imaging Reporting and Data System (BI-RADS) classification (**Box 1**).[4] The BI-RADS assessment guides clinical decision making and the need for biopsy.

Box 1
BI-RADS classification

0: Unsatisfactory assessment; additional imaging needed

1: Negative findings; routine follow-up recommended

2: Benign findings; no malignancy suspected

3: Probably benign lesion; short-term follow-up indicated

4: Suspicious abnormality

5: Highly suggestive of malignancy

6: Known malignancy

Adapted from Sickles EA, D'Orsi CJ, Bassett LW, et al. ACR BI-RADS® mammography. In: ACR BI-RADS® atlas, breast imaging reporting and data system. Reston (VA): American College of Radiology; 2013; with permission.

Solid masses are further evaluated by biopsy. Fine-needle aspiration (FNA) biopsy uses a thin needle that is guided into the mass to remove tissue with or without the use of ultrasound guidance (stereotactic biopsy). FNA biopsy has a high specificity and sensitivity in assessing breast lesions but requires an experienced pathologist to read the results because of the small amount of cells collected.

Core biopsy uses a larger needle than FNA biopsy and removes a small cylinder of tissue. Vacuum-assisted core biopsy takes a larger sample of tissue and is highly effective and accurate. Surgical biopsy removes the entire lesion and a margin of normal-appearing tissue.

BENIGN BREAST MASSES

Benign breast masses are divided into three categories: (1) nonproliferative, (2) proliferative without atypia, and (3) proliferative with atypia. Proliferative BBD with or without atypia is associated with an increased risk of developing breast cancer (**Table 1**).[5–9] Hartman and colleagues[10] found that this increased risk persisted for at least 25 years after initial biopsy. The age at diagnosis of BBD is inversely correlated with risk. Therefore, younger women diagnosed with BBD had an increased risk of breast cancer.

BBD is influenced by hormones with levels of estradiol, estrone, and testosterone higher in women with BBD compared with those without breast pathology. Hormone levels also tend to be higher in women with proliferative disease, compared with those with nonproliferative breast disease. Endometriosis and polycystic ovary syndrome have also been associated with increased risk of BBD, likely caused by altered hormone levels.[11,12]

Nonproliferative Breast Lesions

Breast cysts
Breast cysts are round or ovoid fluid-filled masses that are derived from the terminal duct lobular unit. They are typically firm and mobile, with clear delineation from the surrounding breast tissue. Cysts are a common cause of breast mass in premenopausal women, and are frequently found in women aged 35 to 50.[13] Cysts are uncommon in postmenopausal women who are not on hormonal therapy.[14] A cyst cannot be differentiated from a solid mass on mammogram or clinical breast examination, and ultrasound or FNA is necessary for diagnosis.

Table 1 Breast cancer risk	
Lesion Type:	Risk Ratio
Nonproliferative • Simple cyst • Mild hyperplasia of the usual type	1.27
Proliferative without atypia • Usual ductal hyperplasia • Intraductal papillomas • Radial scars • Simple fibroadenoma	1.88
Atypical hyperplasia • Atypical ductal • Atypical lobular	4.24

Hormonal changes can affect cysts, and they can fluctuate with the menstrual cycle, as well as during periods of hormonal irregularity. Acute enlargement of cysts may cause severe localized pain, and may require drainage of fluid. Simple cysts carry no increased risk for breast cancer.

Complex cysts
Complex cysts have thick walls and/or septa greater than 0.5 mm on ultrasound, and anechoic and echogenic components. A complex cyst should be evaluated by FNA, core biopsy, or excisional biopsy. The malignancy rate is 0.3%, and likelihood of malignancy is increased with ultrasound findings of thickened cyst wall, thick septations, mixed cystic/solid components, and hyperechogenicity.[15]

Mild hyperplasia of the usual type
Mild hyperplasia of the usual type is an increase in the number of epithelial cells within a duct. Epithelial cells are two to four cells in depth, and do not cross the lumen of the involved duct. Diagnosis is made by FNA, core biopsy, or excisional biopsy. Breast cancer risk is not increased.

Proliferative Breast Lesions Without Atypia

Fibroadenomas
Fibroadenomas (FA) are masses of mixed fibrous and glandular tissue that occur in tissue outside of the ducts. These present clinically as a smooth, firm, rubbery well-defined mobile mass, and as a solid mass on ultrasound. FAs are the most frequent cause of a discrete breast lump in young women and occur in 25% of asymptomatic women.[15] Up to 20% of women have multiple FAs in the same breast or bilaterally. They are most commonly found in women aged 15 to 35. FAs occur most often in the upper outer quadrant, and occur in similar frequency in either breast.[16] FAs account for 50% of breast biopsies, and 75% of biopsies in women younger than age 20.[17]

FAs usually form during menarche, and develop from the special stroma of the lobule, not a single cell. The cause is unknown, but is thought to occur as an aberration of normal breast development rather than a benign neoplasm.[16] They do show a hormonal relationship, because they can enlarge during pregnancy or with estrogen therapy, and typically regress during menopause.[17] There has been a direct association between FA and oral contraceptive use before the age of 20, further demonstrating the hormonal relationship.[15]

Definitive diagnosis of FA is by core biopsy or surgical excision. The management of an FA is determined in large part by the patient's age. A significant percentage of lesions undergo spontaneous resolution. Over 1 to 3 years, 16% to 37% of FAs resolve, and 32% resolve by 5 years.[16]

Women younger than age 35 may be managed with short-term sonographic follow-up every 6 months.[17] FAs in young women may also be treated with cryoablation, although only after proven by core biopsy.[18] FAs in women older than age 35 or rapidly growing lesions should be surgically excised.

Many women opt for surgical excision of the mass; however, excision comes with surgical risks including scarring at the incision site, dimpling of the breast from tumor removal, damage to the ductal system, and mammographic changes. Simple FAs have a slightly elevated risk of cancer, with a risk ratio of 1.49.[5]

Complex FAs contain other proliferative changes of the breast including sclerosing adenosis, adenosis, ductal epithelial hyperplasia, epithelial calcifications, or papillary apocrine changes.[5,13,15] Complex FA has an elevated risk of breast cancer (relative risk, 2.27), associated with the histologic features.[5]

Juvenile fibroadenoma

Juvenile FA is most commonly found in adolescents aged 10 to 18 year old, and account for 0.5% to 2% of FAs.[17] These lesions usually present as a unilateral, painless, rapidly growing solitary mass larger than 5 cm. Juvenile FAs can reach 15 to 20 cm. Because of the large size and rapidly growing nature, surgical removal is recommended. Juvenile FAs are benign lesions with no increased risk of breast cancer.

Intraductal papilloma

An intraductal papilloma is a small wart-like growth of fibroglandular tissue that grows into the lumen of the lactiferous ducts. They most commonly occur in women aged 35 to 50 and may present initially as unilateral clear or blood-tinged nipple discharge. Lesions may also be incidentally discovered on mammogram, ultrasound, MRI, or ductogram.

Solitary papillomas are found in the large milk ducts, and are usually felt as a small lump near the nipple. Papillomas in the smaller ducts are often in clusters called multiple papillomas.

Diagnosis is established by core needle biopsy. Although most papillomas are benign, some can harbor areas of atypia or ductal carcinoma in situ. Surgical excision is the standard treatment, but observation with short-term follow-up may be reasonable in a small subset of patients who have papillomas without atypia. Solitary papillomas have no increased risk of breast cancer, but multiple papillomas carry a slightly increased risk.

Usual ductal hyperplasia

Usual ductal hyperplasia is an increase in the number of cells within the duct without architectural changes. Cells may vary in size and shape but remain benign. It is usually found as an incidental finding on biopsy. Risk of future breast cancer is minimal, and no additional treatment is indicated.

Radial scars

Radial scars, or complex sclerosing lesions, are characterized by a fibroelastic core surrounded by radiating ducts and lobules. They are usually found incidentally on breast masses that have been biopsied or excised. Some radial scars may be large enough to be seen on mammography, and may mimic carcinoma. Radial scars may be premalignant lesions, and surgical biopsy is recommended.

Proliferative with Atypia

Atypical hyperplasia

Atypical hyperplasia is a proliferation of dysplastic epithelial cells in either the ducts or the lobules. It is found in approximately 10% of biopsies with benign breast findings. Both atypical ductal hyperplasia and atypical lobular hyperplasia are considered to be premalignant conditions, with a relative risk factor for future breast cancer of 4.24.[10] The cumulative incidence of breast cancer over 25 years is 30%.[9] Timing of the diagnosis of atypical hyperplasia is also a factor, because the younger a woman is at diagnosis, the more likely she is to develop breast cancer in the future.

Diagnosis of atypical hyperplasia is made by core needle biopsy. Once confirmed, surgical excision is recommended. There is a 15% to 30% frequency of upgrading, or chance of finding breast cancer in the case of atypical ductal hyperplasia. In atypical lobular hyperplasia, upgrading rates are 0% to 67%.

Atypical hyperplasia has a two- to four-fold increased incidence of breast cancer compared with a nonproliferative diagnosis. With the significantly increased risk of breast cancer, increased screening may be necessary. Annual screening mammograms and twice-yearly clinical breast examinations are recommended. Currently there are no recommendations supporting the use of MRI for screening after the diagnosis of atypical hyperplasia. Additionally, women should discontinue oral contraceptives, avoid hormone-replacement therapy, and make appropriate lifestyle changes to decrease risk for breast cancer. Chemoprevention of breast cancer using selective estrogen-receptor modulators and aromatase inhibitors may be considered for women with atypical hyperplasia.

OTHER BREAST CONCERNS
Breast Pain

Breast pain, or mastalgia, is a common complaint in women. Pain may be cyclic or noncyclic. Cyclic breast pain typically occurs during the luteal phase of the menstrual cycle and peaks the week before menses. Pain is mediated by hormonal fluctuations of estrogen and progesterone that stimulate proliferation of normal breast tissue. Cyclic breast pain may also be caused by oral contraceptives or other hormonal therapy. Cyclic pain is characteristically bilateral and diffuse.

Noncyclic breast pain is not related to the menstrual cycle and is more likely to be unilateral and focal. Pain may be caused by large breasts, hormone-replacement therapy, mastitis, or abrupt swelling of a cyst. A thorough history and breast examination should be done, and appropriate imaging completed as indicated by examination. Women with classic cyclical pain do not need imaging, although some patients prefer this for their own reassurance.

Breast pain is treated with lifestyle modification, a supportive bra, heat or ice packs, and acetaminophen or nonsteroidal anti-inflammatory drugs. Elimination of caffeine may be helpful for some women, but has not been effective in controlled studies. Likewise, vitamin E and evening primrose oil may alleviate pain in some women, but has been inconclusive in studies. Danazol can be used for more severe mastalgia, but has significant side effects that limit its use.

Breast pain as a presenting symptom of cancer is rare, occurring in only 0.5% to 3.3% of patients. Thus women who present with breast pain and an otherwise normal physical examination have the same risk of breast cancer as women without breast pain.[19]

Lipoma

Breast lipomas are benign solitary tumors that are composed of mature fat cells. They are usually well-circumscribed, soft, nontender masses. Clinical diagnosis of lipoma is confirmed by FNA or core needle biopsy. Surgical excision is indicated if the diagnosis is uncertain or if the lesion grows rapidly. Lipomas do not pose subsequent breast cancer risk.[13,15]

Fat Necrosis

Fat necrosis is a benign condition that occurs secondary to accidental or surgical breast trauma. It may be mistaken for malignancy on clinical breast examination or on mammography, and biopsy may be necessary to confirm diagnosis. Excision of fat necrosis is not needed when confirmed by biopsy, and there is no increased risk of cancer.

SUMMARY

BBD is a common finding in women, the source of which varies significantly and poses variable breast cancer risk. Breast pain, cysts, and FAs can be managed

Table 2
Benign breast lesions at a glance

Lesion	Comments
Breast pain	• Cyclical or noncyclical • Treatment: nonsteroidal anti-inflammatory drugs, supportive bra, danazol • Unlikely to be presenting symptom of cancer
Breast cyst	• Round/ovoid fluid-filled mass • Firm, mobile, well-demarcated • Common in age 35–50
Fibroadenoma	• Mixed fibrous and glandular tissue • Aberration of normal breast development • Smooth, firm, rubbery, mobile mass • Common in age 15–35
Intraductal papilloma	• Wart-like growth in lactiferous ducts • May present with clear or bloody discharge
Ductal hyperplasia	• Increased number of cells in duct without atypia
Radial scar	• Fibroelastic core with radiating ducts and lobules • Found incidentally
Atypical hyperplasia	• Atypical ductal hyperplasia • Atypical lobular hyperplasia • Four-fold increased risk of breast cancer
Lipoma	• Benign tumors of mature fat cells
Fat necrosis	• Occurs after accidental or surgical breast trauma

with observation and short-term follow-up, whereas others, such as intraductal papilloma and atypical hyperplasia, have increased risk for breast cancer, and should be excised. It is also important to consider timing of diagnosis because the cancer risk associated with BBD has an inverse relationship with age, potentially changing the management strategy based on the patient's demographics. Family history of breast disease and breast cancer is also important to consider, particularly in patients with proliferative breast disease with or without atypia because a positive family history does increase the risk of breast cancer in these patients. A firm knowledge of BBD helps women's health providers educate patients and manage the potential risk associated with these common disorders (**Table 2**).

REFERENCES

1. Dyrstad S, Yan Y, Fowler A, et al. Breast cancer risk associated with benign breast disease: systematic review and meta-analysis. Breast Cancer Res Treat 2015;149:569–75.
2. Russo J. Breast development and morphology. 2017. Available at: www.UpToDate.com. Accessed October 25, 2017.
3. Schorge J, Schaffer J, Halvorson L, et al. Breast disease. In: Williams gynecology. New York: McGraw Hill; 2008. p. 269–90.
4. BI-RADS Classification. Available at: www.acr.org. Accessed November 15, 2017.
5. Nassar A, Wisscher D, Degnim A, et al. Complex fibroadenoma and breast cancer risk: a Mayo Clinic benign breast disease cohort study. Breast Cancer Res Treat 2015;153:397–405.

6. Castells X, Domingo L, Corominas J, et al. Breast cancer risk after diagnosis by screening mammography of nonproliferative or proliferative benign breast disease: a study from a population-based screening program. Breast Cancer Res Treat 2015;149:237–44.

7. Tice J, Miglioretti D, Li C, et al. Breast density and benign breast disease: risk assessment to identify women at high risk of breast cancer. J Clin Oncol 2015; 33:3137–43.

8. Worsham M, Raju U, Lu M, et al. Risk factors for breast cancer from benign breast disease in a diverse population. Breast Cancer Res Treat 2009;118:1–7.

9. Samoli E, Trichopoulos D, Lagiou A, et al. The hormonal profile of benign breast disease. Br J Cancer 2013;108:199–204.

10. Hartman L, Sellers T, Frost M, et al. Benign breast disease and the risk of breast cancer. N Engl J Med 2005;353:229–37.

11. Farland L, Tamimi R, Eliassen A, et al. A prospective study of endometriosis and risk of benign breast disease. Breast Cancer Res Treat 2016;159:545–52.

12. Gumus I, Kiktener A, Dogan D, et al. Polycystic ovary syndrome and fibrocystic breast disease: Is there any association? Arch Gynecol Obstet 2009;280:249–53.

13. Sabel M. Overview of benign breast disease. 2017. Available at: www.UpToDate. com. Accessed October 18, 2017.

14. Morrow M. The evaluation of common breast problems. Am Fam Physician 2000; 61(8):2371–8.

15. Guray M, Sahin A. Benign breast diseases: classification, diagnosis, and management. Oncologist 2006;11:435–49.

16. Carty NJ, Ravichandran D, Carter C. Management of fibroadenoma of the breast. Ann R Coll Surg Engl 1995;77:127–30.

17. Greenberg R, Skornick Y, Kaplan O. Management of breast fibroadenomas. J Gen Intern Med 1998;13:640–5.

18. Li P, Xiao-yin T, Cui D, et al. Evaluation of the safety and efficacy of percutaneous radiofrequency ablation for treating multiple breast fibroadenoma. J Can Res Ther 2016;12:C138–42.

19. Golshan M. Breast pain. 2017. Available at: www.UpToDate.com. Accessed October 25, 2017.

Menopause
The Best Chapter of Our Lives

Elyse Watkins, DHSc, PA-C

KEYWORDS

- Menopause • Menopausal transition • Perimenopause • Estrogen
- Vasomotor symptoms • Genitourinary syndrome of menopause

KEY POINTS

- Clinical practice guidelines advise against the use of estrogen solely for the prevention of chronic diseases, such as cardiovascular disease, Alzheimer dementia, and colon cancer.
- Current guidelines advise using the lowest dose of systemic estrogen, if within 10 years of a woman's last menstrual period or before age 60 years, to treat vasomotor symptoms.
- For patients in whom estrogen is not an option, paroxetine is currently the only FDA-approved SSRI for the treatment of vasomotor symptoms; evidence does not support the use of black cohosh, red clover, or soy.
- New pharmacologic treatment options for the genitourinary syndrome of menopause include a DHEA vaginal insert and an oral SERM.
- Patients with a uterus who wish to use estrogen must also take a progestin to help prevent endometrial hyperplasia and uterine cancer, but the addition of a progestin increases the risk of thromboembolic events, dementia, breast cancer, and CVD.

INTRODUCTION

Menopause is clinically defined as the unintentional absence of menses for 1 year because of ovarian senescence resulting in a state of hypoestrogenism. The average age of menopause has remained constant globally at 51 years of age; in contrast, the average age of menarche has declined. Perimenopause is defined as the period of time occurring before a woman's last menstrual period (LMP) where she experiences alterations in sex hormone pulsatility, resulting in menstrual changes.[1] Early perimenopause has a variable duration, but is described as a persistent change in the length of the menstrual cycle of 7 days or more. Pituitary follicle-stimulating hormone (FSH) levels fluctuate during this phase, therefore FSH testing is not recommended to diagnose or stage perimenopause. Late perimenopause is defined as intervals of missed menses equal to or greater than 60 days. Typically, late perimenopause lasts from 1 to

The author has no relationships to disclose.
Department of Physician Assistant Studies, High Point University, One University Parkway, High Point, NC 27268, USA
E-mail address: ewatkins@highpoint.edu

3 years. Menses during late perimenopause are characteristically variable, and sex hormone levels fluctuate considerably.

During early and late perimenopause, anti-Müellerial hormone and inhibin B, both produced by ovarian follicular granulosa cells, remain low. In early postmenopause, FSH levels can again be variable, but at about 6 years after the final LMP, the FSH remains persistently elevated. Transvaginal ultrasounds reveal low antral follicle counts throughout all phases of the menopause transition.

Early postmenopause is divided into three stages (stages +1a, +1b, +1c) based on symptomatology and hormone levels.[1]

- Stage +1a: lasts about 1 year after the final menstrual period; vasomotor symptoms (VMS); FSH variability
- Stage +1b: lasts about 1 year; VMS; FSH variability
- Stage +1c: lasts about 3 to 6 years; variable VMS; FSH remains elevated; estradiol remains low

Late postmenopause occurs approximately 8 years after the final menstrual period. Clinically, women may experience worsening of vulvovaginal atrophy and genitourinary syndrome of menopause (GUSM).[1]

Surgical menopause occurs when the ovaries are removed from a woman premenopausally. Premature ovarian failure, also called primary ovarian insufficiency, is menopause occurring before age 40 years. Many of the somatic and neurocognitive effects of natural menopause occur in surgical menopause and premature menopause. There is evidence that bilateral oophorectomy resulting in surgical menopause is associated with an increased risk of cardiovascular disease (CVD).[2]

THE WOMEN'S HEALTH INITIATIVE

A discussion of hormone therapy must include a brief overview of the Women's Health Initiative (WHI). The WHI, started in 1991 under the auspices of the National Heart, Lung, and Blood Institute, was designed to determine if the use of conjugated equine estrogen and medroxyprogesterone acetate, a progestin, could prevent chronic diseases, such as colon cancer, dementia, and CVD. The initial trial was halted when researchers found a statistically significant increase in cardiovascular events, thrombotic events, and breast cancer. Since then, careful scrutiny of the WHI has revealed several areas of concern regarding methodology, and newer randomized control trials (RCTs) have yielded evidence that has created opportunities for managing VMS, preventing osteoporosis, and treating the GUSM (see **Table 3**).

A SUMMARY OF MANAGEMENT STRATEGIES
Estrogen

Estrogens that are naturally produced in the body are estrone (E1), estradiol (E2), and estriol (E3). Estradiol is the most potent of endogenous estrogens; estriol is found primarily during pregnancy, and estrone during menopause.

There are several synthetic estradiol preparations available in the United States for treatment of menopausal symptoms. Oral estradiol is micronized to help with absorption (**Table 1**).

Phytoestrogens, particularly those found in soy, act as selective estrogen receptor modulators (SERMs). As such, they have the ability to bind to estrogen receptors.[3] Conversion and absorption of phytoestrogens takes place in the human gut. There are vast differences between humans in regards to their gut microbiota. Thus, the bioavailability of phytoestrogens varies considerably from person to person, making

Table 1
Estrogen preparations

Name	Preparations	Comments
Estradiol	Oral, transdermal patch, transdermal gel, transdermal spray, vaginal ring, vaginal tablet, vaginal cream	17-β estradiol
Esterified estrogen	Oral	Metabolized to estrone and estradiol
Estropipate	Oral	Salt of estrone
Ethinyl estradiol	Oral	Commonly used in oral contraceptive pills; much more potent than other estrogen preparations
Conjugated equine estrogens	Oral, vaginal	From pregnant mares' urine; has more than 10 different estrogens
Conjugated synthetic estrogen	Oral	From soy and yam plants; 9 different estrogenic substances

it difficult to predict effectiveness, response, and target tissue binding.[3] The American Association of Clinical Endocrinologists guidelines recommend against the use of soy products in women with a family or personal history of estrogen-dependent cancer, thromboembolism, or CVD.[4]

Xenoestrogens are synthetic compounds that have estrogenic effects and are commonly found in pharmaceuticals, environmental pesticides, some cosmetics, and chemicals used in various industries. Xenoestrogens have been associated with breast cancer and altered reproductive health.[5]

SERMs can act as estrogen agonists or antagonists, depending on the target tissue. A SERM that has antagonist effects on the breast, such as tamoxifen, has agonist effects on the endometrium. Use of tamoxifen is associated with a risk of endometrial hyperplasia. The American College of Obstetricians and Gynecologists (ACOG) recommends that postmenopausal women who take tamoxifen should be screened for endometrial hyperplasia, and that all women should immediately report any vaginal bleeding to their health care provider (**Box 1, Table 2**).[6]

Box 1
Important concepts regarding the use of estrogen

If a woman still has a uterus, she must use a progestin to protect against endometrial hyperplasia if using transdermal or oral estrogen.

Vaginal estrogen use in a woman with an intact uterus does not require a progestin.

Evidence recommends using the lowest possible dose for the shortest amount of time to alleviate menopausal symptoms.

The benefit of estrogen use is likely to outweigh the risks if initiated within 10 years of menopause onset and before age 60 years.

Continuation of estrogen therapy beyond 10 years or after age 60 years is considered only after a careful risk-benefit discussion with the patient and annual re-evaluations.

Vaginal estrogen is initiated at any age.

Compounded estrogen products are not recommended because of lack of Food and Drug Administration oversight and variable potency, purity, and safety data.

Table 2
Examples of SERMs for women

Name	Clinical Use	Agonist/Antagonist
Tamoxifen	Estrogen receptor–positive breast cancer; high risk for developing breast cancer; ductal carcinoma in situ	Agonist on endometrium; antagonist on breast
Raloxifene	Treatment and prevention of osteoporosis in postmenopausal women; risk reduction for invasive breast cancer	Agonist on bone; antagonist on breast, uterus
Bazedoxifene	Combined with conjugated equine estrogen for treatment of vasomotor symptoms in menopause; also used in Europe for treatment and prevention of osteoporosis	Agonist on bone; antagonist on uterus
Ospemifene	Moderate to severe dyspareunia caused by vulvovaginal atrophy in menopause	Agonist on vagina, bone, brain; antagonist on breast

Postmenopausal estrogen use has been associated with breast cancer, thrombotic events, and cardiovascular events, particularly when combined with a progestin. Although transdermal estrogen use has a slightly decreased risk of thrombotic events, careful attention should be paid to established contraindications and precautions for estrogen use (**Box 2**).

Progestogens

Progestins and progesterone are also called progestogens. Progestins are synthetic compounds that have antimitotic effects on the endometrium, reducing the proliferative effect of estrogens. Progestins have been successfully used for type 1 endometrial cancer. Common progestins that are used postmenopausally include norgestimate, norethindrone, and drospirenone. Norgestimate and norethindrone have similar androgenic properties, but drospirenone, a derivative of spironolactone, is antiandrogenic.

Progesterone is a naturally occurring steroid primarily produced by the corpus luteum during a normal menstrual cycle, with a small amount produced by the adrenal glands. Progesterone is antiproliferative on endometrial epithelia. Micronized progesterone is Food and Drug Administration (FDA)-approved; however, the brand name

Box 2
Contraindications and precautions regarding the use of estrogen

Contraindications	Precautions
Personal history of breast and/or uterine cancer	Dyslipidemia (hypertriglyceridemia)
Porphyria	Thrombophilias without a history of thrombotic event
Active liver disease	Migraine headache with aura (transdermal preferred)
Thrombotic disorders	Tobacco use
History of thrombotic event (deep venous thrombosis, pulmonary embolism, cerebrovascular attack)	
Undiagnosed abnormal uterine bleeding	
Transient ischemic attacks	

Prometrium capsules are made with peanut oil, so prescribers are advised to ensure patients do not have a peanut allergy. Contraindications regarding the use of progestins are similar to those for estrogen (**Box 3**).

Testosterone

Testosterone use during menopause has been associated with an overall improvement in sexual function. Testosterone has been reported to have positive effects on bone density and has been associated with decreased depression and anxiety. However, exogenous testosterone can cause hirsutism, acne, an increase in triglycerides, and a decrease in high-density lipoprotein.[7]

No consensus exists regarding the normal testosterone serum level for postmenopausal women. In addition, there is a paucity of well-designed RCTs that assess the risks and benefits of testosterone use in menopause without the addition of estrogen and/or a progestin.

THE IMPACT OF MENOPAUSE ON THE BODY
The Brain

Estrogen is neuroprotective.[8] However, the use of estrogen solely for cognitive benefits in naturally postmenopausal women has not been supported, but some evidence exists for its use after surgical menopause in younger women. There is selected evidence that supports certain mind-body therapies, such as mindfulness-based stress response training and yoga, to help alleviate specific neurocognitive issues associated with menopause.[9]

The use of combination conjugated equine estrogen and medroxyprogesterone acetate in women older than 65 years substantially increases a woman's risk for dementia.[10] The use of conjugated equine estrogen without medroxyprogesterone acetate did not increase a woman's risk of dementia.[10] When estrogen is initiated early in the menopause transition (before age 65 and within 10 years of LMP), there seems to be a decreased risk of Alzheimer dementia.

Box 3
Important concepts regarding progestogens

Progestin and progesterone are distinctly different compounds.

Synthetic progestins are vasoconstrictive and prothrombotic.

Synthetic progestins are used in type 1 endometrial cancer.

Oral micronized progesterone has a favorable lipid effect.

Oral micronized progesterone, instead of a synthetic progestin, may be prescribed to protect the endometrium when using estrogen, but care must be taken to ensure adequate dosing.

Progestins are indicated when a woman has an intact uterus and using systemic estrogen to help prevent endometrial hyperplasia.

Medroxyprogesterone acetate, the progestin used in the Women's Health Initiative Study, has been associated with increased thrombotic events, including stroke.

Use of medroxyprogesterone acetate with conjugated equine estrogens in women more than 20 years postmenopausal is associated with an increase in cardiovascular events.

Medroxyprogesterone acetate has also been linked to an increase in dementia and breast cancer when combined with conjugated equine estrogens.

Several studies have confirmed an objective decline in immediate and delayed verbal recall, verbal fluency, and regional brain activation during the menopausal transition, and sometimes persisting postmenopause.[11,12] It is important to convey to women who present with memory issues that about 5% of Alzheimer disease patients present before age 65.[13]

Approximately 20% of women experience depression during menopause.[14] The later a woman enters menopause, the lower her risk of developing a depressive disorder.[8] Use of estradiol versus other synthetic estrogen products, such as conjugated equine estrogens, has been associated with stronger antidepressant and anxiolytic effects.[15,16] The FDA has approved the use of paroxetine for the treatment of VMS during menopause, so use of this selective serotonin reuptake inhibitor may be of clinical benefit for the treatment of depression and VMS.

The Heart

CVD incidence increases postmenopausally. Pericardial fat accumulation and elevated coronary calcium has been associated with decreased serum estrogen and may be a marker for CVD.[17] Women with surgical menopause have an increased risk of developing CVD earlier than women undergoing natural menopause.[2] Women with early menopause, either surgically induced via bilateral oophorectomy or premature ovarian failure, are at a greater risk of developing CVD, independent of hormone use.[2] Women with an abbreviated reproductive life span of less than 33 years between menarche and menopause experienced statistically significant increased risks of CVD and stroke.[2]

Evidence strongly supports counseling women on the importance of lifestyle choices regarding CVD. Counseling points should include maintaining an active lifestyle, making healthy food choices, tobacco cessation, and limiting alcohol consumption. Screening otherwise asymptomatic women for CVD with electrocardiography is not recommended.[18] Calculated risk-assessment tools are used to assess a woman's overall 10-year risk of developing CVD to help determine if statin therapy is warranted. ACOG guidelines on screening for CVD advises annual testing of blood pressure, fasting glucose, lipids, and a body mass index for women with a history of preeclampsia, but offers no specific guidelines on CVD screening for women without a history of preeclampsia.[19]

Bone

Estrogen therapy reduces the incidence of postmenopausal osteoporotic fractures and prevents bone loss in women with natural and surgical menopause.[10] The combination of conjugated equine estrogen and bazedoxifene is also FDA-indicated for the prevention of osteoporosis in menopausal women.

Weight-bearing, balance, and resistance exercises are recommended to help prevent bone loss and fractures.[20] It may also help prevent sarcopenia. In addition, serum vitamin D_3 levels should be greater than 30 ng/mL, and women should ensure an intake of 1200 mg of calcium every day.[20] ACOG also recommends that postmenopausal women take 600 IU of vitamin D every day.[21] Women need to be counseled to stop smoking tobacco and limit alcohol to two drinks per day. The American Association of Clinical Endocrinologists recommends alendronate, risedronate, teriparatide, denosumab, and zoledronic acid for most patients at high risk of sustaining an osteoporotic fracture via use of the World Health Organization's Fracture Risk Assessment Tool (available for free at http://www.shef.ac.uk/FRAX/index.aspx).

In average-risk women, ACOG recommends a screening dual-energy x-ray absorptiometry scan at age 65.[21] Risks for osteoporosis include tobacco use, weight less than 127 lbs, alcoholism, a parent who sustained a hip fracture, chronic corticosteroid use, and rheumatoid arthritis. For postmenopausal women less than 65 years with risk factors, a screening dual-energy x-ray absorptiometry should not occur more than every 2 years.[21]

In women who are receiving raloxifene for breast cancer risk reduction, and in women using systemic estrogen for VMS, denosumab, teriparatide, or a bisphospho-nate are added in high-risk patients.[20]

Vitamin K has been used in Japan to treat age-related bone loss, but meta-analyses from the United States has revealed mixed results. One small RCT from the Netherlands showed a decrease in bone loss among participants taking vitamin K_2.[22] Currently, there are no evidence-based guidelines to support its use.

Phytoestrogens may be of benefit in the treatment of decreased bone mineral density and osteoporosis, but individual variation in metabolism and conversion make it extremely difficult to standardize treatment. As such, there are no evidence-based recommendations regarding the use of phytoestrogen to treat bone loss in menopause.

CLINICAL PRESENTATION OF MENOPAUSE

The changes most commonly seen in women during the menopause transition include VMS, elongation of the menstrual cycle, and weight gain. Later in menopause, vaginal atrophy may cause dyspareunia and frequent urinary tract infections. Other commonly reported symptoms include decreased libido and sleep disturbance.

Vasomotor Symptoms

VMS, perhaps the hallmark of menopause, occur in up to 85% of patients.[23] Many women have persistent symptoms in to their 70s. The average duration of VMS is 7.5 years.[24,25] ACOG and the North American Menopause Society[10] recommend that women who present with bothersome VMS may use estrogen therapy if the benefits outweigh the risks (see **Boxes 1** and **2**). Newer data suggest that transdermal estrogen may be associated with a decreased risk of thrombotic events compared with oral estrogen; however, the benefit is reduced when a progestin is added to therapy.[26]

The use of phytoestrogens for VMS has revealed mixed results. A recent systematic review and meta-analysis indicated that the use of phytoestrogens can modestly reduce the number of daytime VMS, but not nocturnal VMS, without causing endometrial hyperplasia.[27]

In 2013, the FDA approved the use of paroxetine for moderate-to-severe VMS in menopausal women. Serotonin and norepinephrine reuptake inhibitors, such as venlafaxine and desvenlafaxine, are more effective than placebo, but are not specifically FDA-approved for VMS. Other nonhormonal pharmaceutical options that have been used for VMS include clonidine and gabapentin. Both of these drugs have shown to be more effective than placebo, but concerns regarding side effects have limited their use.

A newer option for women with an intact uterus is the combination of oral conjugated equine estrogen and a SERM, bazedoxifene. Bazedoxifene has antagonist effects on the uterus, therefore, a progestin is not needed.

Other nonhormonal, nonpharmaceutical modalities that have been used for VMS include Gingko biloba, black cohosh, over-the-counter soy products, acupuncture, yoga, and Chinese herbal formulations. There is no evidence that these modalities are more effective than placebo; thus, current practice guidelines do not recommend their use.

Menstrual Changes

Menstrual changes are often one of the first signs of early perimenopause. During early perimenopause, women may experience a change in the length of the menstrual cycle by 7 days or more. During late perimenopause, women may experience intervals of missed menses lasting 60 days or more. One year of unintentional menstrual cessation in the absence of pathology is the hallmark of menopause.

Weight Gain

Postmenopausal women tend to experience body fat distribution changes. Central adiposity increases during the menopause transition and persists postmenopausally.[28] Women should be advised to maintain an active, healthy lifestyle to reduce their overall risks of CVD and type 2 diabetes. It is prudent to follow US Preventive Services Task Force clinical practice guidelines on screening for metabolic disorders, particularly in postmenopausal women.

Sleep

Up to 60% of women in the menopausal transition present with sleep disturbances and insomnia.[29] Nocturnal awakenings occur most frequently, causing decreased sleep efficiency and shorter duration of sleep. The average length of sleep among menopausal women is 6 hours. Most women who experience sleep dysfunction report VMS as a principle cause of nocturnal awakenings.[29] Treatment of VMS with estrogen and selective serotonin reuptake inhibitors may also improve quality of sleep.

Libido

Sexual dysfunction can occur during menopause, particularly if a woman experiences GUSM. Transdermal estrogen, vaginal dehydroepiandrosterone (DHEA), and ospemifene may have a positive secondary effect on low libido. Flibanserin (Addyi), a mixed serotonin agonist/antagonist and dopamine antagonist, is FDA-approved for the treatment of hypoactive sexual desire disorder in premenopausal women only. The FDA has not approved any other treatment modality to treat low libido in women. Mindfulness-based psychological therapies have been used to treat libido issues in women, but large-scale, well-designed RCTs specifically addressed at postmenopausal women have yet to be published.

Genitourinary Syndrome of Menopause

GUSM encompasses vulvovaginal atrophy with subsequent vaginal dryness and burning. Women often experience dyspareunia secondary to atrophy and decreased vaginal lubrication. The atrophic changes in the vagina can also cause symptoms resembling urinary tract infections, such as dysuria, frequency, urgency, and even recurrent infections of the lower urinary tract (**Table 3**).

Table 3	
The genitourinary syndrome of menopause	
Vaginal Dryness	**Urinary Urgency**
Vaginal burning	Urinary frequency
Dyspareunia secondary to decreased vaginal lubrication	Dysuria
Dysorgasmia and/or anorgasmia	Frequent urinary tract infections

Table 4
GUSM pharmacologic treatment options

Pharmacologic Option	Route of Administration	Special Considerations	Progestin Requirement
Estradiol	Vaginal cream, tablet, or ring	If + hx BrCA, consult oncologist	No for the first year; data lacking beyond 1 y
DHEA	Vaginal suppository	Converted into estrogen and androgen	No
Ospemifene	Oral	SERM; agonist on endometrium; need to take with food; Black Box Warning for endometrial CA and CV events	Consider using a progestin because of agonist effects on endometrium

Abbreviations: CA, cancer; CV, cardiovascular.

Localized, topical estrogen is the preferred treatment of GUSM. Evidence supports low-dose vaginal estrogen use without a progestin for menopausal women with GUSM; however, data are not robust regarding endometrial safety beyond 1 year of use.[10]

Newer pharmacologic options include oral ospemifene and an intravaginal DHEA insert, Intrarosa. Fractional CO_2 lasers have been used with success in small RCTs and remain a viable option for patients where the use of any estrogen is contraindicated or those who may not tolerate topical estradiol or DHEA therapy (**Table 4**).

SUMMARY

Since the WHI, there has been increased research about the effects of estrogen and progestins on a menopausal woman's body, with professional medical societies reframing their clinical practice guidelines to reflect the state of the evidence. There are also new approaches to treating the neurocognitive and somatic effects of menopause, making it vital that PAs who care for women during the menopause transition and are postmenopausal should stay apprised of pharmacologic and nonpharmacologic options for treatment.

REFERENCES

1. Harlow SD, Gass M, Hall JE, et al. Executive summary of the stages of reproductive aging workshop + 10: addressing the unfinished agenda of staging reproductive aging. J Clin Endocrinol Metab 2012;97(4):1159–68.
2. Ley SH, Li Y, Tobias DK, et al. Duration of reproductive life span, age at menarche, and age at menopause are associated with risk of cardiovascular disease in women. J Am Heart Assoc 2017;6:e006713.
3. Lagari VS, Levis S. Phytoestrogens for menopausal bone loss and climacteric symptoms. J Steroid Biochem Mol Biol 2014;13:294–301.
4. Goodman NF, Cobin RH, Ginzberg SB, et al. American Association of Clinical Endocrinologists medical guidelines for clinical practice for the diagnosis and treatment of menopause. Endocr Pract 2011;17(6):1–25. Available at: https://www.aace.com/files/menopause.pdf.
5. Farooq A. Structural and functional diversity of estrogen receptor ligands. Curr Top Med Chem 2015;15(4):1372–84.

6. American College of Obstetricians and Gynecologists. Committee opinion: tamoxifem and uterine cancer. Number 601. 2014. Available at: https://www.acog.org/Resources-And-Publications/Committee-Opinions/Committee-on-Gynecologic-Practice/Tamoxifen-and-Uterine-Cancer. Accessed November 29, 2017.

7. Elraiyah T, Sonbol MB, Wang Z, et al. The benefits and harms of systemic testosterone therapy in postmenopausal women with normal adrenal function: a systematic review and meta-analysis. J Clin Endocrinol Metab 2014;99(10):3543–50.

8. Georgakis MK, Thomopoulos MD, Diamantaras A-M, et al. Association of age at menopause and duration of reproductive period with depression after menopause: a systematic review and meta-analysis. JAMA Psychiatry 2016;73(2): 139–49.

9. Woods NF, Mitchell ES, Schnall JG, et al. Effects of mind-body therapies on symptom clusters during the menopausal transition. Climacteric 2014;17(1): 10–22.

10. The NAMS 2017 Hormone Therapy Position Statement Advisory Panel. The 2017 hormone therapy position statement of the North American Menopause Society. Menopause 2017;24(7):728–53.

11. Epperson CN, Sammel MD, Freeman EW. Menopause effects on verbal memory: findings from a longitudinal community cohort. J Clin Endocrinol Metab 2013; 98(9):3829–38.

12. Berent-Spillson A, Persad CC, Love T, et al. Hormonal environment affects cognition independent of age during the menopause transition. J Clin Endocrinol Metab 2012;97(9):E1686–94.

13. Zhu XC, Tan L, Wang H-F, et al. Rate of early onset Alzheimer's disease: a systematic review and meta-analysis. Ann Transl Med 2015;3(3):38.

14. Cohen LS, Soares CN, Vitonis AF, et al. Risk for new onset of depression during the menopausal transition: the Harvard study of moods and cycles. Arch Gen Psychiatry 2006;63(4):385–90.

15. Hiroi R, Weyrich G, Koebele SV, et al. Benefits of hormone therapy estrogens depend on estrogen type: 17-β estradiol and conjugated equine estrogens have differential effects on cognitive, anxiety-like, and depressive-like behaviors and increase trypthophan roxylase-2 mRNA levels in dorsal raphe nucleus subregions. Front Neurosci 2016;10:517.

16. Gleason CE, Dowling NM, Wharton W, et al. Effects of hormone therapy of cognition and mood in recently postmenopausal women: findings from the randomized, controlled KEEPS-Cognitive and Affective Study. PLoS Med 2015;12: e1001833.

17. El Khoudary SR. Postmenopausal women with greater paracardial fat have more coronary artery calcification than premenopausal women: the study of Women's Health Across the Nation (SWAN) Cardiovascular Fat Ancillary Study. J Am Heart Assoc 2017;6(2) [pii:e004545].

18. United States Preventive Services Task Force. Coronary heart disease: screening with electrocardiography. Available at: https://www.uspreventiveservicestaskforce.org/Page/Document/UpdateSummaryFinal/coronary-heart-disease-screening-with-electrocardiography. Accessed November 29, 2017.

19. American College of Obstetricians and Gynecologists. High-risk factors. Available at: https://www.acog.org/About-ACOG/ACOG-Departments/Annual-Womens-Health-Care/Well-Woman-Recommendations/High-Risk-Factors. Accessed November 29, 2017.

20. Camacho PM, Petak SM, Binkley N, et al. American Association of Clinical Endocrinologists and American College of Endocrinology clinical practice guidelines

for the diagnosis and treatment of postmenopausal osteoporosis 2016. Endocr Pract 2016;22(Suppl 4):1–42. Available at: https://www.aace.com/files/postmen opausal-guidelines.pdf. Accessed November 29, 2017.

21. American College of Obstetricians and Gynecologists. Practice bulletin no. 129: osteoporosis. Obstet Gynecol 2012;120(3):718–34.

22. Knapen MHJ, Drummen NE, Smit E. Three-year low-dose menaquinone-7 sup-plementation helps decrease bone loss in healthy postmenopausal women. Os-teoporos Int 2013;24:2499–507.

23. Thurston RC, Jofee H. Vasomotor symptoms and menopause: findings from the study of women's health across the nation. Obstet Gynecol Clin North Am 2011;38(3):489–501.

24. Avis NE, Crawford SL, Greendale G, et al. Study of women's health across the Nation. Duration of menopausal vasomotor symptoms over the menopause tran-sition. JAMA Intern Med 2015;175:531–9.

25. The American College of Obstetricians and Gynecologists. Practice bulletin no. 141: management of menopausal symptoms. Obstet Gynecol 2014;123(1): 202–16.

26. American College of Obstetricians and Gynecologists. Committee opinion: post-menopausal estrogen therapy: route of administration and risk of venous throm-boembolism. Number 556, 2013. Available at: https://www.acog.org/Resources-And-Publications/Committee-Opinions/Committee-on-Gynecologic-Practice/Postmenopausal-Estrogen-Therapy. Accessed November 29, 2017.

27. Franco OH, Chowdhury R, Troup J, et al. Use of plant-based therapies and meno-pausal symptoms: a systematic review and meta-analysis. JAMA 2016;315(23): 2554–63.

28. Donato GB, Fuchs SC, Oppermann K, et al. Association between menopause status and central adiposity measured at different cutoffs of waist circumference and waist-to-hip ratio. Menopause 2006;13(2):280–5.

29. Baker FC, Willoughby AR, Sassoon SA, et al. Insomnia in women approaching menopause: beyond perception. Psychoneuroendocrinology 2015;60:96–104.

Female Sexual Interest and Arousal Disorder

How We Can Help When Our Patient's Libido Hits the Brakes

Nisha McKenzie, PA-C, CSC, IF

KEYWORDS

- Female sexual dysfunction • Hypoactive sexual desire disorder
- Female sexual interest and arousal disorder • Low libido
- Comprehensive treatment approach • Sexual pain • Sexual health
- Sexuality counseling

KEY POINTS

- Female sexual interest and arousal disorder is a reality for many women, yet is underdiagnosed and undertreated.
- It has recently been recognized that, although most studies cite more than 40% of women will express concern regarding sexuality, a smaller subset are likely distressed by the issue.
- Research is beginning to look at distress as a necessary factor in diagnosing female sexual interest and arousal disorder. Further research will help in development of treatment options, inclusive of counseling techniques and pharmacotherapy.

INTRODUCTION

Sexuality is a vital aspect of human life, recognized and used in countless different ways. It can wax and wane throughout different time periods and life events, but can be distressing if desire remains low despite a change in circumstances. Low sexual desire is the most common sexual difficulty experienced by women.

When low desire persists and becomes distressful, female sexual interest and arousal disorder (FSIAD) could be the diagnosis. The following is a brief synopsis regarding how to recognize this disorder and how to progress if it is diagnosed.

Disclosure Statement: The author currently has a financial relationship as an independent contractor/speaker with AMAG Pharmaceuticals.
Women's Health, Center for Women's Sexual Health, Grand Rapids OB/GYN, 5060 Cascade Road Suite C, Grand Rapids, MI 49546, USA
E-mail address: nisham@grandrapidsobgyn.com

FEMALE SEXUAL DYSFUNCTION

Female sexual dysfunction (FSD) is an umbrella term encompassing all aspects of pain, orgasm, desire, and sexual response. Unlike male sexual dysfunction, FSD remains relatively unstudied with few commercially available treatment options. There is complex interplay of psychological, social, cultural, physiologic, and religious undertones to FSD making it difficult for anyone who specializes in any one of those areas to feel competent in treating the disorder.

HYPOACTIVE SEXUAL DESIRE DISORDER AND FEMALE SEXUAL INTEREST AND AROUSAL DISORDER

Hypoactive sexual desire disorder (HSDD) is the subset of FSD that focuses on desire, the most prevalent of the FSDs. It was first defined in the Diagnostic and Statistical Manual of Mental Disorders (DSM) in 1987. The definition has changed several times to date. In 2013, the DSM-V[1,2] was released and has combined HSDD with Female Sexual Arousal Disorder and named it Female Sexual Interest and Arousal Disorder (FSIAD) (see DSM-IV[2] and DSM-V criteria for FSD). It is presently defined by the DSM-V as the absence of or significant reduction in sexual interest/arousal for at least 6 months. Three of the following symptoms must also be present:

- Absent/reduced interest in sexual activity
- Absent/reduced sexual/erotic thoughts/fantasies
- No/reduced initiation of sexual activity; unresponsive to partner's attempt to initiate
- Absent/reduced sexual excitement/pleasure during sexual activity in at least 75% of encounters
- Absent/reduced sexual interest/arousal in response to any internal or external sexual/erotic cues (eg, written, verbal, visual)
- Absent/reduced genital or nongenital sensations during sexual activity in at least 75% of sexual encounters

FSIAD can be classified as generalized or situational, lifelong or acquired, and mild, moderate, or severe in distress. In other words, if a woman has been distressed by her level of sexual interest for greater than 6 months, but goes on vacation with her partner and finds herself in a sea of erotic bliss, she is not likely to have a diagnosis of generalized FSIAD, but rather situational FSIAD.

The problem must also cause clinically significant distress. It must not be better explained by a nonsexual mental disorder, severe relationship distress or other stressors, or effect of a substance/medication or another medical condition.

A critical diagnostic criterion is the element of distress. It is interesting to note that although a certain level of communication or sexual frequency can be distressing to one woman, the same scenario in another woman may feel healthy. No quantitative diagnostic tool exists for FSIAD, only the level of distress caused by the dysfunction.

PREVALENCE

Studies assessing the impact of low sexual desire have varied widely in endpoints over the years. The difficulty with comparison of data lies in the lack of notation of distress in the previous DSM-IV-TR criteria. A study sampling 741 women across Australia, the Americas, Europe, and Asia reported the prevalence of problems with sexual desire varied from 3.0% to 31.0%. They were evaluated using DSM-IV-TR-IV criteria for HSDD as well as a validated questionnaire.[3] The WISHeS study also used validated questionnaires and the DSM-IV-TR criteria, thus also not inclusive of distress, and found the range to be between 9% in naturally postmenopausal women and 26% in younger surgically postmenopausal women.[4]

Only recently have studies begun to investigate the prevalence of FSIAD in relation to distress, which is now required for diagnosis. Results from the PRESIDE study, the largest US study to date to survey female sexual problems associated with distress, reveals that of more than 30,000 respondents the prevalence of any sexual problem was 43.1% and sexually related personal distress was reported at a level of 22.2%.[5] The British National Survey of Sexual Attitudes and Lifestyles produced similar findings, noting 34.2% of women reported lacking interest in sex; distress was included in this study as well.[6]

CONTRIBUTING FACTORS

Many medical conditions and numerous medications as well as cigarette smoking can negatively affect sexuality, partially accounting for the varied estimates regarding prevalence (**Table 1**).

In addition to medical conditions, relational patterns of communication affect partner interactions as well as the cultural, spiritual, and religious messages received during adolescence and beyond. The interplay of the physiologic, psychological, and social aspects of a sexual disorder can render previously held communication patterns ineffective.

Physician assistants are uniquely positioned to help their patients by normalizing the stigma around discussions of sexuality. Many patients will not ask, but are hoping that the topic is brought up during their visit.[34] Discussion surrounding many of these myths, not only for healthcare providers (HCP) but also for patients, will help dispel the stigma surrounding healthy sexuality. **Table 2** highlights some of the many reasons sexuality lacks transparency in the medical setting.

HISTORY

A thorough history is integral to making an appropriate diagnosis and developing a specific and beneficial management plan for patients who are afflicted with FSD.

Table 1 Contributing factors to sexual dysfunction	
Medical Conditions	**Medications**
Diabetes[7–10]	Antipsychotics[28]
Coronary artery disease[11]	SSRI[29,30]
Hypertension[12,13]	Tricyclic antidepressants
Hypothyroidism or hyperthyroidism[14]	Chemotherapeutic agents
Congestive heart failure	Aromatase inhibitors
Seizure disorder	Triglyceride-lowering agents
Depression[15–17]	Histamine receptor (H2) blockers
Musculoskeletal/movement disorders[18–20]	Weight loss medications
Chronic pain	Antiepileptics
Genital pain	Immunosuppressants
Substance abuse	Central α-adrenergic agonists
Hormonal disruptions[21,22]	β-Blockers
Endocrine disorders[23]	Diuretics
Arthritis[24]	GnRH agonists
Incontinence: urinary or fecal[25,26]	Oral contraceptives[31–33]
Cancer[27]	

Table 2	
Reasons sexuality remains unspoken of in medical clinics	
Reasons HCPs Do Not Discuss	**Reasons Patients Do Not Discuss**
Lack of sufficient training[34]	Fear of judgment
Fear of embarrassment/misunderstood	Fear of embarrassment
Lack of known referral resources	Social norms/expectations ("good" girls shouldn't
Time constraints	want more sex)
Lack of knowledge regarding	Insurance won't cover such concerns
reimbursement	Lack of awareness of FSIAD
Belief that patient appears happy and	Lack of awareness regarding treatment options
healthy so no need to ask	Told by another HCP that it is normal
	Fear their HCP will try to "fix" their sexuality
	(expression, interest, identity)
	Fear of job loss/discrimination based on sexual
	practices

The following are key steps to facilitate obtaining a complete and accurate sexual health history.

- *Ask with her clothes on.* Allow her to remain clothed during the history-taking portion of the visit. Answering questions regarding sexual health can be scary, but allowing her to remain clothed will help her feel some level of control and increased comfort.
- *Avoid assumption.* Discuss sexual health with every patient starting at the age of 11 with no ending age. Avoid the assumption that someone is not sexually active based on age, medical status, relationship status, or anything else.
- *Assure confidentiality.* Feeling safe is essential for disclosure of sensitive topics relating to sexual health. Verbalize your commitment to her privacy and to her wellness.
- *Normalize.* Let her know that "as your caregiver, comprehensive health is my primary concern. In that, I ask all of my patients about sexual health."
- *Possible referral point.* If her response feels uncomfortable or unfamiliar to you, now is a good time to make a referral.
- *Match her vocabulary.* If you choose to continue the conversation, meet your patient at her level with vocabulary. Using terms unfamiliar to her will cause a greater divide in the room. If your patient uses a term you are unfamiliar with, ask her what she means. Show her that you are listening and ready to learn from her. This includes her use of pronouns. If unsure, ask every time as identity and sexuality can change.
- *Open with ubiquity-style questions.* This will help normalize potential concerns and will have a higher yield than direct questions. Such statements as "Many women, while breastfeeding, experience vaginal dryness or pain as well as issues with lowered sex drive. How has this been for you?" will allow her to feel more comfortable in disclosing this information as well as less alone in her struggle.
- *Silence.* This is a difficult one! We are accustomed to directing conversations and maximizing our time in the examination room. However, it is important to remember that you may have just asked her a question that no one has ever brought up, and one that may have been weighing on her for some time. She may go through an internal, albeit quick, process of thoughts before answering:
  - No one has asked me that before.
  - How did they know?
  - Did my provider just say the word orgasm?

- ○ Do I out myself?
- ○ Do I trust this provider
- ○ Will my insurance pay for this?
- ○ What can they do anyway?
- ○ I've never told this to anyone.
- ○ Will I be betraying my partner by telling my provider?
- ○ What if they know one of my friends and tell them?
- *Possible referral point*. If her response after the silence is outside your comfort level, now is a good time to reaffirm normality and refer.
- *Follow with specific questions*. Otherwise, once she has responded with a sexual concern, then follow with more specific questions such as, "Are you having difficulty with orgasm?" "Is lubrication a concern for you?" "Are you noticing a decrease in your motivation for sex?" These specific questions will help differentiate between different clinical subtypes of FSIAD.
- *Follow-up positive response with more open-ended questions*. "Tell me more about that."
- *Possible referral point*. Multiple points in this process can serve as referral points, depending on experience and comfort level.
- *Assess patient goals*. By the end of the visit, be sure to ask her to relay her goal to you, remembering it may be different from what you think her goal should be. Verbalizing a goal will set realistic expectations and allow for more accurate assessment of her response to treatment.

Time is essential in medicine, so HCPs can ask and refer immediately, or counsel to their comfort level. It is not the HCP's responsibility to have been taught all the nuances of the human body. It is their responsibility to know what resources are available to enhance care for each of the patients.

EVALUATION

Although many women request hormonal testing to help evaluate potential causes of decreased libido, this is recommended in a select few. A start should be with a comprehensive medical, relationship, and sexual history to help customize the workup for each patient. If a genital examination is indicated, as in cases of FSD related to sexual pain or endocrine changes, the vulva, vagina, pelvic floor, uterus, and adnexa should be fully evaluated. Many screening tools are also available to help the busy clinician assess patients for necessary workup and the need for follow-up (**Table 3**).

Laboratory examination is necessary only when there is reasonable expectation that results will affect the treatment plan. Premature menopause is one example that would require laboratory workup to define.

COUNSELING

Utilization of the PLISSIT model (*P*ermission, *L*imited *I*nformation, *S*pecific *S*uggestions, *I*ntensive *T*herapy) of sex therapy is a helpful tool to bridge the gap with information between permission and intensive therapy. This model was created in 1976 by Jack S. Annon to guide HCPs through the levels of evaluation and treatment.[39] Assessment is broken down into the following 4 core steps:

- *Permission*: First, create an environment where the patient feels comfortable revealing concerns, assuring confidentiality and using either open-ended or ubiquity style questions.

Table 3
Screeners for hypoactive sexual desire disorder/female sexual interest and arousal disorder

Screening Tool	Assessment
Decreased Sexual Desire Screener	Brief diagnostic tool for HSDD. Sensitivity and specificity 84% and 88%, respectively[35]
Female Sexual Function Index	19-item, self-report scale considered gold-standard measure of female sexual function. Assess domains of desire, arousal, orgasm, pain[36]
Female Sexual Distress Scale-Revised	Distress[37]
Sexual Interest and Desire Inventory-Female	Clinician administered tool to measure severity and change in response to treatment of HSDD[38]

- *Limited Information*: Second, offer limited information based on the history taken and the concern presented. This information could include discussion of the bio-psychosocial model of sexual health and the multiple causes for the concern or basic genital anatomy. This type of counseling can educate and empower your patient, thereby dispelling potentially long-held myths and misconceptions regarding sexuality.[40]
- *Specific Suggestions*: Next, specific suggestions may be made, including offering a differential diagnosis. This portion of PLISSIT is whereby HCPs may exercise latitude to determine the extent of counseling performed based on level of comfort or experience with the topic. Recommendations could include the use of specific lubricants or moisturizers for dryness, massage, vibration, dilators, or bibliotherapy. Education on benefits of self-stimulation as well as diet, exercise, stress-reduction, and social norms can positively impact sexual health. Discussions may also include the differences between female and male sexual response cycles, the importance of communication skills, reciprocity and transparency in sexual wants and needs, the use of fantasy, and different ways to achieve orgasms. It may be necessary to normalize self-stimulation and educate regarding techniques, timing, and discussion with partner. Many women are uncomfortable or unfamiliar with the use of a vibrator. Framing the use of vibration in a medical sense, in that it will increase blood flow to an area to assist in tissue health and healing, much like using a vibrating massage wand on a shoulder spasm, can help normalize this process for many women and speed healing.

Insertional pain due to many disorders, such as vulvovaginal atrophy (whether this be due to menopause, breastfeeding, or use of oral contraceptives), lichen sclerosus, vaginismus, and many forms of vulvodynia can benefit from increased touch. Counsel regarding the importance of massage and again liken this to massage of a neck spasm. Increased blood flow to any tissue will speed healing. Massage and vibration are both methods of increasing blood flow to the neck or to the vulva. Specific instructions will help with compliance. If possible, have demonstration vibrators on hand in the clinic to let women see and touch them, thus decreasing fear of the potentially unknown. Using a pelvic floor model, demonstrate specific massage techniques, applying gentle pressure between the thumb and forefinger to massage and stretch the tissue. She may incorporate this massage technique while applying topical medication or moisturizer. Write down instructions regarding technique, pressure, and frequency.

If you feel comfortable, you could introduce techniques such as sensate focus. Sensate focus is a sex therapy technique initially defined by Masters and Johnson, although since refined.[41] This technique works on removing the goal-oriented nature of many sexual encounters and helps remind participants of the joy of being intimate with a partner. It takes penetration off the table for an agreed on amount of time while the couple works on experiencing touch and the many benefits of being mindful of sensations other than strictly genital sensations.

- *Intensive Therapy*: If there is need for referral to other specialists, namely for intensive therapy, this can be made at this point as well.

TREATMENT

Approach to treatment requires acknowledgment of the biopsychosocial aspects of human sexuality.[42] Not to say that HCPs need to be experts in each of these areas, but to say that it is imperative to recognize there are typically multiple contributing factors. The ability to relay this recognition to the patient will also help establish reasonable goals and expectations throughout the course of treatment, thereby increasing compliance and satisfaction. Increased understanding of the process will also aid them in following through with referrals to other specialists who can help address the many factors involved.

PHARMACOTHERAPY
Flibanserin

Flibanserin (Addyi) is the only US Food and Drug Administration (FDA) -approved pharmacotherapeutic agent available for HSDD and is indicated for acquired, generalized HSDD or FSIAD of any severity in premenopausal women. Flibanserin is a $5-HT_{1A}$ agonist/$5-HT_{2A}$ antagonist that also exhibits weak to moderate antagonism of $5-HT_{2B}$, $5-HT_{2C}$, and dopamine D4 receptors. Approved in August 2015, it fell short of hype and expectations. It was widely referred to in the media as the female Viagra, leading people to expect an immediate, visible response to this medication. However, this is a centrally acting central nervous system agent taken nightly before change is noted within approximately 8 weeks. Cost, lack of awareness, and the FDA-mandated Risk Evaluation and Mitigation Strategy (REMS) program make this medication difficult to access for most patients. The dual control model of sexual response involves a teeter totter of inhibitory mechanisms and excitatory mechanisms.[43] The excitatory hormones dopamine and norepinephrine, and the inhibitory neurotransmitter serotonin, are proposed to balance with the use of Flibanserin.

The REMS program does pose another barrier to obtaining this medication. Prescribers are required to take a short, 10-minute, 4-question test before being certified to prescribe Flibanserin. Pharmacies also need to take the test before dispensing. Because this was implemented due to findings on the study of Flibanserin with alcohol, it requires the prescriber to evaluate the alcohol study. It is important to note that typical alcohol use was allowed during the studies to approve Flibanserin, and approximately 60% of women admitted to social alcohol use during the study period.[44]

The initial alcohol study was performed in 25 participants; 23 of these participants were men. After a 10-hour fast, participants were fed a light breakfast and instructed to take Addyi (this is intentionally dosed at bedtime) with either 2 or 4 of the following: 12-oz cans of beer with 5% alcohol content, 5-oz glasses of wine with 12% alcohol content, or 1.5-oz shots of 80-proof spirit. Hypotension or syncope requiring thera-peutic intervention of ammonia salts and/or placement in supine or Trendelenburg po-sition occurred in 4 of the 23 subjects coadministered Flibanserin 100 mg and 2 of each of the alcoholic beverages. Six of the subjects coadministered Flibanserin and 4 of the alcoholic beverages experienced orthostatic hypotension when standing from a seated position, and 1 of the 6 required therapeutic intervention.[45] This study design creates debate regarding the REMS program, applicable clinical evidence, and gender bias in sexual research.

A separate, larger alcohol study including women was completed October 2016 but is not yet published. Two further alcohol studies are also currently underway.

The difficulty in predicting the efficacy of Flibanserin in each patient lies within the complexities of the biopsychosocial model of FSD. Each aspect is weighted differ-ently in every patient. Some patients will require more psychosocial work; others will require more biological work. Most, however, will require some combination of both.

Those patients who are not good candidates for, or do not respond to, Flibanserin are left with off-label medications or hormone supplementation if warranted. Because of the relative lack of on-label options, many medications have been studied and used off label for the treatment of HSDD/FSIAD.

Testosterone

Testosterone is produced in both the ovaries and the adrenal glands. Beginning just before the age of 30, testosterone levels begin a slow, steady decline and decrease dramatically after either surgical or natural menopause. Just as the menopausal symp-toms of hot flashes and night sweats do not manifest in every woman after the decline of estrogen, decreased libido may not manifest in every woman with a decrease in testosterone. This fact is one of many factors rendering the success of testosterone therapy in women a difficult endpoint to assess. However, there are multiple studies showing efficacy of testosterone supplementation in both premenopausal and post-menopausal women for the treatment of HSDD. In fact, testosterone use in women has been studied with increasing frequency in recent years. Although still not FDA approved, off-label testosterone use has shown efficacy in clinical trials in women who are surgically menopausal and treated with estrogen and progesterone, surgically and naturally menopausal not treated with estrogen and progesterone, and premenopausal.[46–50]

Many providers are apprehensive to use testosterone in premenopausal women because of concerns regarding virilization as well as potential androgenic effects on the fetus in the case of pregnancy. Thirty-four premenopausal women with low libido and low testosterone levels were evaluated in a 12-week study using 1% testosterone cream, 10 mg applied daily to the thigh, and showed improvement in well-being, mood, and sexual function.[51]

Testosterone can be administered in many different forms: oral, transdermal, in-jections, or implants. However, the use of testosterone in women with HSDD re-mains quite controversial, with some studies showing efficacy, and others highlighting potential side effects. Nonetheless, testosterone has been used in women with symptoms of androgen deficiency since 1930. Despite the lack of conclusive evidence regarding the long-term effects of testosterone use in women, there is little doubt in the literature that it does help improve the female sexual response.

Because testosterone is not FDA approved for use in women, there remains little guidance regarding dosing, counseling, and monitoring. Although it is generally recommended that providers regularly observe women for signs of virilization, the American Association of Clinical Endocrinologists has offered monitoring guidelines for women using testosterone supplementation. Recommendations include semiannual clinical breast examinations along with annual mammography, lipid panel, complete blood count, and endometrial sonography. Some experts also recommend baseline and regular testing of calculated free testosterone.[52]

Androgenic side effects may be seen, such as acne, hirsutism, deepening of the voice, enlarging of musculature, or enlarging of clitoris. These effects, however, are typically only seen at supraphysiologic doses.[53] Although there is a lack of data regarding long-term cardiovascular effects, no significant effects have been demonstrated on the lipid panel, fasting glucose, insulin, liver function, or blood counts in women.[47]

Bupropion

Bupropion can also be used off-label in selective serotonin reuptake inhibitors (SSRI) -induced sexual dysfunction. A double-blinded sham-controlled study demonstrated an increase in sexual frequency and desire as compared with placebo after administration of Bupropion (150 mg twice a day). The women in this study were diagnosed with SSRI-induced sexual dysfunction using a validated questionnaire.[54] These findings have been repeated in multiple studies finding success with either the addition of Bupropion to the SSRI or the substitution of Bupropion for the SSRI.

Buspirone

Buspirone is another centrally acting medication that modulates the excitatory and inhibitory pathways involved in sexual response. It may be used as an off-label adjunct for HSDD as well, despite limited safety and efficacy data.[55]

Sildenafil

In postmenopausal women, sildenafil has shown improvements in vaginal lubrication and clitoral sensitivity, but has not proven to be effective at increasing overall sexual function.[56] Female sildenafil users with FSD secondary to multiple sclerosis, diabetes, or antidepressant use, however, note a small, but significant improvement in sexual function.[57]

Combination Therapy

A recent study shows promising effects with the use of combination therapy with testosterone and buspirone or testosterone and sildenafil. This study showed an increase in satisfying sexual events (SSE), although it did not measure distress.[58]

What's on the Horizon?

Society is beginning to recognize the importance of female sexual health as a subset of overall health. As such, further studies are being conducted to help increase understanding regarding cause as well as treatment options for HSDD/FSIAD. As these studies are completed, medications are being studied and developed that may have positive effects on female sexuality. **Table 4** lists upcoming medications currently under review with the FDA for the treatment of FSD.

Table 4
What's on the horizon in sexual medicine

Drug Name	Drug Component(s)	Pharma Sponsor	Approval Status
Lybrido (on demand oral tablet)	Sildenafil + Testosterone	Emotional Brain	Phase III for HSDD
Lybridos (on demand oral tablet)	Buspirone + Testosterone	Emotional Brain	Phase III for HSDD
Tefina (intranasal testosterone gel)	Testosterone	Trimel Pharmaceuticals	Phase II complete for anorgasmia
Lorexys (daily oral combination)	Trazadone + Bupropion	S1 Biopharma	Phase IIa complete for HSDD
Rekynda (Bremelanotide) (on demand subQ injection)	Melanocortin agonist	AMAG Pharmaceuticals and Palatin Technologies	2 Phase III trials completed for HSDD/FSIAD, coprimary endpoints met

SUMMARY

Sexuality has long been a culturally taboo topic of discussion and to this day remains misunderstood and often misrepresented. As physician assistants, we have made a commitment to improve the overall health of our patients. This commitment is not possible while excluding sexual health. Our best avenue to this end is to further our own knowledge regarding the possibilities surrounding human sexuality and to be aware of our own preconceived notions, experiences, and biases. Once we understand the vast complexities of human relationships, our judgments begin to pale and our minds begin to open. This space is where we can best offer comprehensive, nonjudgmental, empathic, and informed health care to each patient we have the honor to treat.

REFERENCES

1. American Psychiatric Association. Diagnostic and statistical manual of mental disorders: DSM-V. Arlington (TX): American Psychiatric Publishing; 2013.
2. American Psychiatric Association. Diagnostic and statistical manual of mental disorders: DSM-IV-TR. 4th edition. Arlington (TX): American Psychiatric Publishing; 2000.
3. McCabe MP, Goldhammer DL. Prevalence of women's sexual desire problems: what criteria do we use? Arch Sex Behav 2013;42(6):1073–8.
4. Leiblum SR, Koochaki PE, Rodenberg CA, et al. Hypoactive sexual desire disorder in postmenopausal women: US results from the Women's International Study of Health and Sexuality (WISHeS). Menopause 2006;13(1):46–56.
5. Shifren JL, Monz BU, Russo PA, et al. Sexual problems and distress in United States women: prevalence and correlates. Obstet Gynecol 2008;112(5):970–8.
6. Graham CA, Mercer CH, Tanton C, et al. What factors are associated with reporting lacking interest in sex and how do these vary by gender? Findings from the third British national survey of sexual attitudes and lifestyles. BMJ Open 2017; 7(9):e016942.
7. Enzlin P, Mathieu C, Vanderschueren, et al. Diabetes and female sexuality: a review of 25 years' research. Diabet Med 1998;15:809–24.

8. Schreiner Engel P, Schiavi RC, Vietorisz D, et al. The differential impact of diabetes type on female sexuality. J Psychosom Res 1987;31:23–33.

9. Erol B, Tefekli A, Ozbery I, et al. Sexual dysfunction in type II diabetic females: a comparative study. J Sex Marital Ther 2002;28(1):55–62.

10. Enzlin P, Mathieu D, VanDenBruel A, et al. Prevalence and predictors of sexual dysfunction in patients with type 1 diabetes. Diabetes Care 2003;26:409–23.

11. Salonia A, Briganti A, Montorsi P. Sexual dysfunction in women with coronary artery disease. Int J Impot Res 2002;14(4):80–92.

12. Okeahialam BM, Obeka NC. Sexual dysfunction in female hypertensives. J Natl Med Assoc 2006;98:638–78.

13. Burchardt M, Burchardt T, Anastasiadis AG, et al. Sexual dysfunction is common and overlooked in female patients with hypertension. J Sex Marital Ther 2002;28:17–26.

14. Salonia A, Lanzi R, Nappi RE, et al. Sexual dysfunction in dysthyroidal women. Int J Impot Res 2002;14(4):52–60.

15. Kennedy SH, Dickens SE, Eisfeld BS, et al. Sexual dysfunction before antidepressant therapy in major depression. J Affect Disord 1999;56:201–9.

16. Frohlich P, Meston C. Sexual functioning and self-reported depressive symptoms among college women. J Sex Res 2002;39:321–6.

17. Bartlik B, Kocsis JH, Legere R, et al. Sexual dysfunction secondary to depressive disorders. J Gend Specif Med 1999;2:52–60.

18. Sipski ML, Alexander CJ. Sexual activities, response and satisfaction in women pre- and post-spinal cord injury. Arch Phys Med Rehabil 1993;74:1025–34.

19. Hennessey A, Robertson NP, Swinger R, et al. Urinary fecal and sexual dysfunction in patients with multiple sclerosis. J Neurol 1999;246:1027–59.

20. Yu M, Roane DM, Miner CR, et al. Dimensions of sexual dysfunction in Parkinson disease. Am J Geriatr Psychiatry 2004;12:221–7.

21. Davis SR, Davison SL, Donath S, et al. Circulating androgen levels and self-reported sexual function in women. JAMA 2005;294:91–7.

22. Dennerstein L, Dudley EC, Hopper JL, et al. Sexuality hormones, and the menopausal transition. Maturitas 1997;26:83–92.

23. Davis SR, Guay AT, Shifren JL, et al. Endocrine aspects of female sexual dysfunction. J Sex Med 2004;1:82–8.

24. Panus RS, Mihailescu GD, Gomisiewicz MT, et al. Sex and arthritis. Bull Rheum Dis 2000;49:1–4.

25. Shaw C. A systematic review of the literature on the prevalence of sexual impairment in women with urinary incontinence and the prevalence of urinary leakage during sexual activity. Eur Urol 2002;42:432–72.

26. Salonia A, Zanni G, Nappi RE, et al. Sexual dysfunction is common in women with lower urinary tract symptoms and urinary incontinence: results of a cross-sectional study. Eur Urol 2004;45:642–50.

27. Wettergren L, Kent EE, Mitchell SA, et al. Cancer negatively impacts on sexual function in adolescents and young adults: the AYA HOPE study. Psychooncology 2017;26(10):1632.

28. Krebs M, Leopold K, Hinzpeter A, et al. Current schizophrenia drugs: efficacy and side effects. Expert Opin Pharmacother 2006;7:1005–21.

29. Gregorian RS, Golden KA, Bahce A, et al. Antidepressant induced sexual dysfunction. Ann Pharmacother 2002;36:1577–666.

30. Clayton AH. Female sexual dysfunction related to depression and antidepressant medications. Curr Womens Health Rep 2002;2:182–9.

31. Warnock JK, Clayton A, Croft H, et al. Comparison of androgens in women with hypoactive sexual desire disorder: those on combined oral contraceptives (COCs) vs. those not on COCs. J Sex Med 2006;3:878–960.
32. Bancroft J, Hammond G, Graham C. Do oral contraceptives produce irreversible effects on women's sexuality? J Sex Med 2006;3:567–639.
33. Wallwiener M, Wallwiener LM, Seeger H, et al. Effects of sex hormones in oral contraceptives on the female sexual function score: a study in German female medical students. Contraception 2010;82:155–64.
34. Bitzer J, Giraldi A, Pfaus JA. Standardized diagnostic interview for hypoactive sexual desire disorder in women: standard operating procedure (SOP Part 2). J Sex Med 2013;10(1):50–7.
35. Clayton AH, Goldfischer ER, Goldstein I, et al. Validation of the decreased sexual desire screener (DSDS): a brief diagnostic instrument for generalized female hypoactive sexual desire disorder (HSDD). J Sex Med 2009;6:730–8.
36. Rosen R, Brown C, Heiman J, et al. The Female Sexual Function Index (FSFI): a multidimensional self-report instrument for the assessment of female sexual function. J Sex Marital Ther 2000;26:191–208.
37. Derogatis LR, Rosen R, Leiblum S, et al. The Female Sexual Distress Scale (FSDS): initial validation of a standardized scale for assessment of sexually related personal distress in women. J Sex Marital Ther 2002;28:317–47.
38. Sills T, Wunderlich G, Pyke R, et al. The Sexual Interest and Desire Inventory-Female (SIDI-F): item response analyses of data from women diagnosed with hypoactive sexual desire disorder. J Sex Med 2005;2(6):801–18.
39. Annon JS. The PLISSIT model: a proposed conceptual scheme for the behavioral treatment of sexual problems. J Sex Educ Ther 1976;2(1):1–15.
40. Bitzer J, Brandenburg U. Psychotherapeutic interactions for female sexual dysfunction. Maturitas 2009;63:160–3.
41. Weiner L, Avery-Clark C. Sensate focus in sex therapy: the illustrated manual. New York: Routledge, Taylor & Francis Group; 2017.
42. Bitzer J, Giraldi A, Pfaus J. Sexual desire and hypoactive sexual desire disorder in women. Introduction and overview. Standard Operating Procedure (SOP Part 1). J Sex Med 2013;10(1):36–49.
43. Bancroft J, Graham CA, Janssen E, et al. The dual control model: current status and future direcdtions. J Sex Res 2009;46(2–3):121–42.
44. Thacker H, Fugh-Berman A, Hirsch A. Should OB/GYNs prescribe Flibanserin for their patients? A look at the pros and cons of this new drug for women with low sexual desire. Contemp Ob Gyn 2016;61(8):34.
45. Stevens DM, Weems JM, Brown L, et al. The pharmacodynamic effects of combined administration of flibanserin and alcohol. J Clin Pharm Ther 2017;42(5):598–606.
46. Shifren JL, Davis SR, Moreau M, et al. Testosterone patch for the treatment of hypoactive sexual desire disorder in naturally menopausal women: results from the INTIMATE NM1 Study. Menopause 2006;13:770.
47. Shifren JL, Braunstein GD, Simon JA, et al. Transdermal testosterone treatment in women with impaired sexual function after oophorectomy. N Engl J Med 2000;343:682–8.
48. Buster JE, Kingsberg SA, Aguirre O, et al. Testosterone patch for low sexual desire in surgically menopausal women: a randomized trial. Obstet Gynecol 2005;105:944.
49. Braunstein GD, Sundwall DA, Katz M, et al. Safety and efficacy of a testosterone patch for the treatment of hypoactive sexual desire disorder in surgically

menopausal women: a randomized, placebo-controlled trial. Arch Intern Med 2005;165:1582.
50. Simon J, Braunstein G, Nachtigall L, et al. Testosterone patch increases sexual activity and desire in surgically menopausal women with hypoactive sexual desire disorder. J Clin Endocrinol Metab 2005;90:5226.
51. Goldstat R, Briganti E, Tran J, et al. Transdermal testosterone therapy improves well-being, mood, and sexual function in premenopausal women. Menopause 2013;10:390–8.
52. Wierman M, Basson R, Davis S. Androgen therapy in women: society clinical practice guideline. J Clin Endocrinol Metab 2006;91(10):3697–710.
53. Margo K, Winn R. Testosterone treatments: why, when and how? Am Fam Physician 2006;73(9):1591–8.
54. Clayton A, Warnock J, Kornstein S, et al. A placebo-controlled trial of bupropion SR as an antidote for selective serotonin reuptake inhibitor-induced sexual dysfunction. J Clin Psychiatry 2004;65(1):62–7.
55. Goldstein I, Kim NN, Clayton AH, et al. Hypoactive sexual desire disorder: International Society for the Study of Women's Sexual Health (ISSWSH) expert consensus panel review. Mayo Clin Proc 2017;92(1):114.
56. Kaplan S, Reis R, Kohn I, et al. Safety and efficacy of sildenafil in postmenopausal women with sexual dysfunction. Urology 1999;53(3):481–6.
57. Schoen C, Bachmann G. Sildenafil citrate for female sexual arousal disorder: a future possibility? Nat Rev Urol 2009;6(4):216.
58. Tuiten A, van Rooij K, Bloemers J, et al. Efficacy and safety of on-demand use of 2 treatments designed for different etiologies of female sexual interest/arousal disorder: 3 randomized clinical trials. J Sex Med 2018;15(2):201–16.

Human Immunodeficiency Virus and Pregnancy

Perinatal Transmission, Medication Management, Monitoring, and Delivery Options

Stephanie P. Elko, MSPAS, PA-C[a],*, Erin McCartney, MPAS, PA-C[b]

KEYWORDS

- HIV • Pregnancy • Perinatal HIV transmission • Antiretroviral therapy • Prenatal care
- HIV replication cycle • CDC and Rutgers François-Xavier Bagnoud Center task force

KEY POINTS

- This article reviews HIV pregnancy testing guidelines and HIV diagnosis in pregnancy, followed by recommended perinatal monitoring of mother infected with HIV and the fetus.
- Understanding the process of perinatal HIV transmission occurs and how to prevent transmission is discussed in this article.
- This article outlines task force goals to eliminate perinatal HIV transmission.
- Discussion of the HIV replication cycle in relation to perinatal transmission prevention and antiretroviral therapy option for during pregnancy takes place within this article.
- This article also outlines the antiretroviral therapy and pregnancy recommendations for antenatal, intrapartum, and postpartum for women infected with HIV. These approaches are further broken down into treatment naive, or patients who have never been on antiretroviral therapy; those who have previously been on therapy but are not currently; and those currently receiving therapy.

INTRODUCTION

At the end of 2014, there were approximately 1.1 million people living with human immunodeficiency virus (HIV).[1] Of these 1.1 million, some of their infections may have resulted from transmission during the perinatal period or via breastfeeding, whereas others were acquired from behaviors. Adding close to 4 million live births in 2015, the potential for pregnancies occurring with an HIV-infected mother becomes

No disclosures to state for S.P. Elko or E. McCartney.
[a] Physician Assistant Studies, Augsburg University, 2211 Riverside Avenue, Campus Box 149, Minneapolis, MN 55454, USA; [b] Division of Maternal Fetal Medicine, Eastern Virginia Medical School, 825 Fairfax Avenue, Suite 310, Norfolk, VA 23507, USA
* Corresponding author.
E-mail address: stephanie.elko@gmail.com

Physician Assist Clin 3 (2018) 399–410
https://doi.org/10.1016/j.cpha.2018.02.008
2405-7991/18/© 2018 Elsevier Inc. All rights reserved.

evident.[2] Approximately 8500 women living with HIV give birth annually, but this is based on an estimate last given in 2006.[3] In all, this is likely a medical condition that most providers come across at some point in their career.

The annual rate of perinatal acquired HIV infection has decreased drastically in the United States, from 3.6 per 100,000 in 2008 to 1.8 per 100,000 in 2013. Unfortunately, this rate differs based on ethnicity, and although the rates among African American perinatal acquired HIV infections also have decreased, the decrease was from 12.7 per 100,000 to 7.1 per 100,000, which is still slower than women of other ethnicities.[4] Through all of the statistics and numbers, it is important to recognize that although strides have been made in decreasing rates of HIV transmission, there is still room for improvement.

HUMAN IMMUNODEFICIENCY VIRUS PERINATAL TRANSMISSION PREVENTION

Transmission from mother to child is the most common cause of childhood HIV. Transmission can occur in utero by the HIV crossing the placenta, by vertical transmission during vaginal delivery, or through breastfeeding via breast milk. Since the 1990s, there has been a decline of more than 90% of perinatal mother-to-child transmissions due to advancements in HIV research, treatment, and prevention.[5] These advancements have included the recommendation that all women, and their partners, considering pregnancy be offered HIV screening. According to the Centers for Disease Control and Prevention (CDC) all women who are, or are considering, pregnancy be screened for HIV infection. If the preconception testing confirms a positive diagnosis of HIV, patients, along with their partners and their health care providers, should discuss starting antiretroviral therapy (ART) as early as possible. This recommendation, called pre-exposure prophylaxis, helps decrease fetal transmission, thus protecting mothers and their offspring and reducing perinatal complications.[5]

The CDC and Rutgers François-Xavier Bagnoud Center have created a task force with a goal of eliminating mother-to-child transmission in the future. Several prevention challenges have been identified, and tools to address these challenges have been created and initiated (**Table 1**).[5]

GENERAL APPROACH TO THE HUMAN IMMUNODEFICIENCY VIRUS PREGNANT PATIENT

Knowing the nature of HIV and its accompany morbidities the general patient's health, it is apparent that women with HIV infection who become pregnant need comprehensive and continuous monitoring throughout pregnancy, and ideally beyond. The approach should be multifaceted for both mother and fetus. The mother should have routine prenatal care, including office visits, general screenings, and routine ultrasound evaluation, as well as undergo regular surveillance of laboratory testing, including but not limited to, CD4 T-lymphocyte (CD4) counts, viral load measurements, drug-resistance testing, antiretroviral (ARV) drug level monitoring, coinfection screening, and sexually transmitted infection testing.[6] Patients should also be monitored for opportunistic infections throughout pregnancy, particularly for toxoplasmosis and cytomegalovirus. Serologies for these infections are recommended for pregnant HIV patients given the high risk and often delayed diagnosis.[6] Furthermore, inquiring about and monitoring for high-risk behaviors, such as continued drug use, is recommended. If these behaviors are present, intervention and referral should be initiated as soon as possible.[7]

According to the CDC, all pregnant women should be screened for hepatitis B virus (HBV) early in each pregnancy. In pregnant women with HIV infection, however,

Table 1	
Centers for Disease Control and Prevention and Rutgers François-Xavier Bagnoud Center HIV and pregnancy challenges and plans to address	
Centers for Disease Control and Prevention Noted Prevention Challenges	**Centers for Disease Control and Prevention Plans to Address**
Pregnant women with HIV may not know they are infected.	Recommend HIV testing for all women as part of routine prenatal care. AMA creating a new CPT code to include HIV testing in prenatal testing on obstetric panel.
Many HIV medical care providers do not have the specialized expertise to address preconception care, family planning services, or prenatal care for women living with HIV.	CDC and François -Xavier Bagnoud Center created an expert panel with goal of best practices and operational guidelines for providers.
Women living with HIV may not know they are pregnant, how to prevent or safely plan a pregnancy, or what they can do to reduce the risk of transmitting HIV to their baby.	Routine health care visits, take medications as directed, ensure infants receive their HIV medications, avoid breastfeeding, and avoid prechewing others', including children's, food.
The risk of perinatal HIV transmission is much higher if a mother's ARV HIV treatment is interrupted at any time during pregnancy, labor, or delivery or if HIV medicines are not provided to her infant.	Provide education regarding possible pregnancy symptoms and medication side effects with patient, and offer treatment option plans. Also provide consistent medical care.
Social and economic factors, especially poverty, affect access to all health care and disproportionately affect people living with HIV.	Address all patient barriers, including improving access to medical care, and providing substance abuse treatment, behavioral health treatment, and access to shelter.

Abbreviations: AMA, american medical association; CPT, current procedural terminology.
Data from HIV among pregnant women, infants, and children. CDC.gov. 2017. Available at: https://www.cdc.gov/hiv/group/gender/pregnantwomen/index.html. Accessed November 11, 2017.

coinfection screening is recommended and includes hepatitis C virus and tuberculosis screening for each pregnancy, unless a coinfection has already been diagnosed.[8] Furthermore, if a woman screens negative for HBV, she should receive the HBV vaccination series during pregnancy. Data have not shown harm to the developing fetus by the HBV vaccination series. To proceed with the HBV vaccination, the CD4 count should be greater than 10 IU/mL.[8] The women who have coinfections of HBV should be consulted by infectious disease. Their ART should incorporate medications that are active against both HIV and HBV.[8] Women with HIV and a coinfection with hepatitis C virus follow the same HIV management as those without HCV coinfection. Current data do not support the use of anti-HCV therapy medications during pregnancy.[8]

Ideally, the maternal and fetal prenatal care should also include referral to infectious disease and high-risk obstetric or maternal-fetal medicine specialties as available. All patients should be recommended for counseling, given the potentially overwhelming demands of pregnancy and HIV care.[7] Perinatal discussion should take place, including maternal and fetal complications, risks, medication side effects and risks, plans for labor and delivery (including the option of cesarean section to reduce maternal-fetal transmission), and recommendations against breastfeeding due to the transmission rate.[7]

HUMAN IMMUNODEFICIENCY VIRUS MEDICATION MANAGEMENT DURING PREGNANCY

Women infected with HIV who become pregnant have an increased risk of perinatal complications, in some cases regardless of viral load.[9] These complications can often be drastically reduced with the appropriate implementation of ART. If ART is appropriately monitored, it is generally well tolerated and with minimal toxic side effects.[10] There are several approaches to treating HIV in a perinatal patient. To better understand the process of ART, however, the process of the HIV life or replication cycle first must be understood.

Human Immunodeficiency Virus Replication Overview

During the HIV replication process, HIV is invading and destroying a host's CD4 T lymphocytes and multiplying the virus. The HIV replication process can be broken down into the following steps: (1) entry (binding and fusion), (2) reverse transcription, (3) integration, (4) replication (transcription and translation), (5) assembly, and (6) budding and maturation (**Fig. 1**).[11]

Entry is the process that involves the binding of HIV to the CD4 cells. On binding, the membrane is promoted to fusion and internalization of the HIV genetic material and enzymes needed for further replication.[11] Next, reverse transcription occurs. Here HIV uses reverse transcriptase to convert HIV RNA into DNA. The double-stranded DNA molecule travels to the CD4 lymphocyte nucleus. Once in the nucleus, the virus uses the enzyme integrase to integrate its double-stranded DNA into the CD4 cell's DNA, which is termed, *integration*. At this point, the CD4 cell has the viral DNA for the remainder of its life. The replication process follows integration. During this process, HIV uses the host CD4 cell material to replicate the HIV RNA, which is translated into new viral particles.[11] Next comes the assembly of these new viral particles, mainly made up of HIV proteins and enzymes. Together these particles migrate from the nucleus to the cell's outer membrane, where they are assembled into an immature, noninfectious HIV package, or bud. The final step is release of the HIV bud from the CD4 cell's outer membrane. On release the viral enzyme, protease, cleaves the HIV polyprotein chains into smaller, functional viral proteins. These matures into infectious HIV particles, and the process repeats itself.[6,11]

General Guidelines for Antiretroviral Therapy During Pregnancy

HIV maternal-fetal transmission rate can be reduced to less than 2% in areas that have the capacity to administer widespread ART.[7,10] ART should be initiated as soon as possible to reduce transplacental transmission and thus reduce HIV-related perinatal complications. Data have shown that ARV medications cross the placenta, which reduces the potential of transplacental HIV transmission.[7] There has also been documentation that ART is associated with preterm delivery and lower birth weights than the general population.[7,10,12] That said, there are known and well-documented benefits of treating HIV-infected pregnant women, and the bottom line is that all pregnant women infected with HIV should be treated with ART because benefits outweigh the risks.[7,12]

Not all ART regimens have been created equal. The provider must consider all the benefits and risks, including overall patient health status, comorbidities, HIV viral load, viral resistance profile, medication adverse effects, drug interactions, and a patient's ability to adhere to the medication regimen.[7,10,12,13] Furthermore, the provider must consider the pregnancy risks. ARV medications are generally placed in 4 categories: preferred (known risks), alternative (higher side-effect risk), insufficient data to recommend the drug, or not recommending the drug.[13] These medications fall into 6

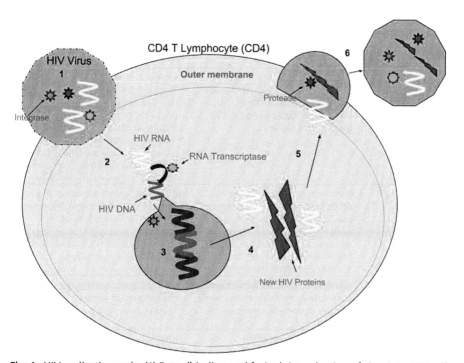

Fig. 1. HIV replication cycle. (1) Entry (binding and fusion): introduction of virus into CD4 cell. (2) Reverse transcriptase: release of viral RNA and use of RNA transcriptase to convert to DNA. (3) Integration: incorporation of viral DNA into CD4 cell DNA via integrase enzyme. (4) Replication: creation of HIV RNA and proteins via the CD4 cell DNA. (5) Assembly: assembly of HIV proteins, enzymes, and RNA into immature HIV, which are noninfectious. (6) Budding: release of immature HIV from CD4 cell with cleaving of proteins by protease. These cleaved proteins combine to form mature HIV, which can infect other cells. (*Data from* The HIV life cycle. Understanding HIV/AIDS. 2017. Available at: https://aidsinfo.nih.gov/understanding-hiv-aids/fact-sheets/19/73/the-hiv-life-cycle. Accessed November 11, 2017; and Overview of antiretroviral agents used to treat HIV. UpToDate.com. 2017. Available at: https://www.uptodate.com/contents/overview-of-antiretroviral-agents-used-to-treat-hiv?source=search_result&search=hiv%20treatment%20adult&selectedTitle=3~150#H14340701. Accessed November 24, 2017.)

ART categories, based on their mechanism of action (**Table 2**). Further delineation occurs at the patient level and depending on the patient has had previous treatment. This is the level at which the ART regimen decisions occur.[8–13] The 3 main approaches are as follows:

1. ART-naive patients
2. Patients previously treated with ART who are not currently being treated
3. Patients currently on ART medications

ARV medications are often used in combination with each other. Generally, the approach to therapy is with 3 agents.[11] The most commonly used ART medication category is nucleoside/nucleotide reverse transcriptase inhibitors (NRTIs), which are considered the backbone of HIV treatment. There are several medications and medication combinations within this category. A second category is the non-NRTI (NNRTIs). These are often used in conjunction with NRTIs and have several

Table 2
Antiretroviral therapy categories and use in general HIV patients and pregnant HIV patients

Medication	General HIV Patient Use	HIV Pregnant Patient Use
NRTIs	Used routinely in HIV patients, commonly given as dual therapy, with some coformulated medication. Can be used in the general HIV patient.	Favored as dual therapy in conjunction with either a PI or INSTI as a 3-drug regimen. Possible concerns of preterm birth have not been concluded. Preferred agents: tenofovir disoproxil fumarate-emtricitabine or tenofovir disoproxil fumarate-lamivudine; abacavir-lamivudine
NNRTIs	Often used in conjunction with NRTIs with several generations of medication; early generations used for drug-naive patients, whereas later generations used for drug-resistant virus. Monitor for mitochondrial toxicity.	Alternative agent: efavirenz and rilpivirine (limited data). Efavirenz can be used with dual-NRTI backbone therapy. Monitoring of mental health status is indicated; exacerbation may occur.
INSTIs	Commonly considered a third agent for treatment-naive patients; used in conjunction with nucleoside analogs	Preferred agent: raltegravir Nonpreferred agents: dolutegravir and elvitegravir
FIs	Used for patients who are treatment-experienced and not been exposed to medication previously; only approved agent is enfuvirtide	Enfuvirtide not recommended; limited pregnancy data
PIs	Able to be used in combination with nucleosides or as anucleoside-sparing or limited regimen; often needs administration with boosting agent medication	Preferred agents: ritonavir-boosted atazanavir, ritonavir-boosted darunavir. Nonpreferred agent are PIs boosted with cobicistat.
CCR5 antagonists (entry inhibitors)	Patients with treatment-experience and drug-resistant virus; maraviroc only approved agent	Only continue if successful for patient; limited pregnancy data
Pharmacologic boosters	Additional medication that increase the efficacy of the ARV medication	See above.

Data from Refs.[10,11,15]

generations. Early NRTI generations are used for drug-naive patients, whereas the later generations are used for drug-resistant virus. A third category is the integrase strand transfer inhibitors (INSTIs), which are commonly considered a third agent for treatment-naive patients. They are used in conjunction with nucleosides analogs. Fourth, are fusion inhibitors (FIs), which are used in regimens of treatment-experienced patients that have not been exposed to FIs previously. Fifth are protease inhibitors (PIs), which have the ability to be used in combination with nucleosides or as a nucleoside-sparing or limited regimens. Often PIs need administration with a boosting agent. Boosting agents help improve the initial drug potency. Lastly, are CCR5 antagonists. These drugs work as entry inhibitors and are used with patients who are treatment-experienced and have a drug-resistant virus.[7–14]

If a woman with known HIV becomes pregnant and is stable and virally suppressed on her ARV regimen, she should remain on that same regimen without interruption or discontinuation.[12] Regardless of which of the categories the patient falls into, the provider must also be aware that pregnancy may alter the pharmacokinetics and medication levels, and viral loads must be monitored throughout the pregnancy.[10] If after 4 weeks to 6 weeks a woman has not achieved appropriate viral suppression, further investigation is warranted. This is completed first by obtaining a medication adherence history, then considering drug-resistance testing, and lastly the creation of a new ART regimen.[10]

Current Antiretroviral Therapy Regimens for the Pregnant Patient with Human Immunodeficiency Virus

Antiretroviral therapy–naive patients

If a patient has a new diagnosis of HIV during pregnancy, there are several options of medication regimens. A patient should be started on a complete 3-drug regimen; however, there are combination pills as well. It is recommended to have 2 NRTIs combined with a PI or integrase inhibitor.[13] For simplicity reasons, only a few examples are discussed in this article. One option includes tenofovir disoproxil fumarate-emtricitabine (Truvada) once daily and raltegravir (Isentress) twice daily. Tenofovir disoproxil fumarate-emtricitabine contains 2 NRTIs and raltegravir is the integrase inhibitor—making this a successful regimen. Another option includes taking tenofovir disoproxil fumarate-emtricitabine, as discussed previously, once daily; atazanavir (Reyataz), once daily; and ritonavir (Norvir), once daily. This second option contains 2 NRTIs, but this time a PI that is Norvir boosted, which is important because it helps assure viral suppression more than Reyataz alone. Norvir has a boosted dose recommendation in pregnancy. A third option is abacavir-lamivudine (Epzicom); atazanavir (Reyataz), once daily; and ritonavir (Norvir), once daily. This regimen includes 2 different NRTIs, abacavir-lamivudine (Epzicom), and a PI with a boosting agent, ritonavir (Norvir).[13]

Antiretroviral therapy in treatment-experienced patients

Patients who were previously treated for HIV infection but are not currently on ART need a thorough medication history as well as drug-resistance testing and baseline virology laboratory tests. Based on these findings an ART regimen can be chosen, ideally with the pregnancy-preferred ARV agents. If these agents have been or are shown to be resistant, then it is appropriate to initiate an alternative agent regimen.[10,13]

Currently on antiretroviral therapy regimen patients

Patients currently on an ARV regimen with good viral suppression and toleration of medications should continue that regimen even if ARV medications are not considered pregnancy-preferred agents. There are few exceptions to this rule.[12] One of 2 exceptions is treatment with didanosine (Videx), stavudine (Zerit), or dose-related (not boosted regimens) ritonavir (Norvir).[13] These 3 medications should be discontinued due to risk of toxicity during the pregnancy, not to be confused with teratogenicity. No drug regimen should be discontinued due to teratogenicity concerns, because prior studies have refuted ARV medications as an outright cause of birth defects.[14] The second exception came out in November 2017 regarding elvitegravir-cobicistat, which is an integrase inhibitor. Elvitegravir-cobicistat was noted to have loss of drug levels during pregnancy, which can lead to loss of virologic suppression.[10]

Special Considerations of Antiretroviral Therapy

Women who are prescribed PIs during pregnancy may need early screening for gestational diabetes. This is important because the PIs have been linked to hyperglycemia. This must also be kept in mind when prescribing for women with preexisting diabetes, because it can exacerbate diabetes and has even been linked to diabetic ketoacidosis.[13]

Women taking zidovudine-containing drugs require routine complete blood cell counts for hematologic changes. These drugs have been known to cause hematologic toxicity and profound anemia in some HIV patients.[8,11] Women using tenofovir in their regimens need closer monitoring of renal function due to toxicity, whereas reverse transcriptase inhibitor medications have been linked to hepatic steatosis and lactic acidosis in pregnancy.[8] Lastly, if any patients are placed on abacavir-containing regimens, such as Epzicom, they must first be tested for the HLA-B*5701 allele. If they are positive, they are at risk for a hypersensitivity reaction and should not be placed on that regimen.[13]

BASIC MONITORING OF THE HUMAN IMMUNODEFICIENCY VIRUS PATIENT DURING PREGNANCY

Pregnancy is a time of body taxation, and, with an infection, such as HIV, and its treatment, the taxation can be life-threatening if not properly managed. All HIV-infected pregnant women should have routine monitoring of liver function testing, serum urea nitrogen and creatinine, and complete blood cell count with differential. They also need monitoring of the HIV RNA levels, or viral load, and CD4 counts. The viral load can be correlated with the risk of HIV maternal-fetal transmission. When the viral load reaches less than 200 copies/mL, a patient is believed to have successfully reached viral suppression.[8] Upon ART, it is recommended that the HIV viral loads have a decline of at least 1 log by the end of the first month and ideally complete suppression by 16 weeks to 24 weeks.[8,15] Drug resistance is generally defined when the HIV viral load is greater than 500 copies/mL to 1000 copies/mL.[15]

The provider should assess the CD4 counts at the first prenatal visit and recheck at least every 3 months.[15] ARV medications have the potential to become toxic to the patient and potentially the pregnancy. Protecting pregnant women with decreased CD4 counts is of particular importance if the counts become less than 200 cells/mm³. At that point, women should be placed on *Pneumocystis jirovecii* pneumonia prophylaxis. The first-line treatment recommendation is with trimethoprim (TMP)-sulfamethoxazole (SMX).[8,13,15] According to *Drugs in Pregnancy and Lactation*, 10th edition by G. Briggs et al[16] TMP has a pregnancy category of "Human and Animal Data Suggest Risk" and SMX has "Human Data Suggest Risk in 3rd Trimester." Alternative treatment options are dapsone or atovaquone, both categorized as "Compatible- Maternal Benefit >>> Embryo/Fetal Risk."[16] A risk and benefit patient discussion must also take place, which should include the taking the risks of prophylactic medications versus the risk of a serious opportunistic infection. Furthermore, glucose-6-phosphate dehydrogenase (G6PD) testing must be completed for both TXP-SMX and dapsone use. If the CD4 count is less than 50 cells/mm³, prophylaxis for disseminated *Mycobacterium avium* complex must also be considered with azithromycin.[8,13,15] Another opportunistic infection that can be suppressed with the use of TMP-SMX is *Toxoplasmosis gondii*, which should be screened for in HIV-infected pregnant women during routine obstetric screenings due to high infection risk. If a woman is positive for toxoplasmosis, she must be placed on suppression treatment if the CD4 cell counts become less than 100 cells/μL.[15] It is also prudent to watch the laboratory tests for anemia and elevated liver function test results, in particular aspartate aminotransferase/alanine aminitransferase.[13] Pregnancy can cause these issues and ART can compound the risks.[13]

Monitoring and management of HIV-infected pregnant women also includes routine fetal assessment with ultrasound. Data have shown an increased association of low birthweight and/or small for gestational age in women treated with ART.[15] An ultrasound should ideally be performed early in the first trimester for accurate dating and during the second trimester for a full fetal anatomy evaluation.[8] This is not due to the concerns of ART on fetal development but rather the continued research of newer ARV medications during pregnancy.[15] During the third trimester, it is important to routinely monitor for fetal growth, with both fundal height and ultrasound as needed.

Routine vaccinations for HIV-infected women should follow the same guidelines as for non–HIV-infected pregnant women. Women with HIV, however, should also receive pneumococcal and hepatitis A and hepatitis B vaccination series.[15]

Special consideration should be given to HIV-infected pregnant patients having significant morning sickness, because this can severely affect compliance with their ART. Open dialogue is important at every visit, because missing doses can contribute to viral resistance over time.[5]

OVERVIEW OF INTRAPARTUM MANAGEMENT

Delivery modes should be considered for all women who are pregnant and infected with HIV. Generally, if a woman has been compliant with her ART regimen and has achieved viral suppression, the transmission of HIV from mother to fetus is low during delivery regardless of route of delivery. Current guidelines quantify a low transmission risk as maternal HIV viral loads, near the time of delivery, as undetectable or less than or equal to 1000 copies/mL. Conversely, high transmission risk is linked to patients with maternal HIV viral load of greater than 1000 copies/mL near the time of delivery or those who did not use ART.[8,10,17] Both of the high-risk groups are recommended to have delivery by caesarean section at 38 weeks or as soon as possible if no antepartum ART was used.[8,10,17] In addition, intrapartum ART should be initiated immediately for these high-risk groups.[17] During delivery, all HIV patients should be started on intravenous zidovudine at 2 mg/kg dose followed by a continuous infusion of 1 mg/kg/h until delivery, given for 3 hours prior to caesarean section, as well as continued on their routine ARV therapies, if applicable.[10,17] All obstetric intrapartum care should aim to minimize the exposure of fetal and maternal fluids exchange to decrease the risk of transmission.[17]

BASIC POSTPARTUM MANAGEMENT

On delivery, or within hours of delivery, all neonates with HIV-infected mothers should receive ART to decrease the risk of the infant acquiring HIV infection. The drug choices should be based on the mother's HIV status.[10] This approach can be further broken down by maternal viral load, less than 1000 copies/mL or greater than 1000 copies/ mL. If the mother had sufficient suppression on delivery, the risk of acquisition of HIV to the infant is low. Conversely, if the mother did not receive, or achieve, sufficient viral suppression, the infant has a higher risk of acquiring HIV and thus should be treated with a 2-ART to 3-ART approach. The therapies are generally recommended to continue for 6 weeks.[10] During this time, infants need close monitoring for drug toleration and safety.

During the postpartum period, the mother should also continue her ART. A strong emphasis on adherence is needed during this time, because studies suggest a decreased compliance in the postpartum period, especially with a lack of social support.[10,18] Therapy may also be modified at this time for optimal suppression, adherence, and treatment of the patient, without the added concern of pregnancy outcomes. HIV-infected women should have received counseling and be ready to begin birth control early in the postpartum period.[5,17,18]

In addition to the recommendations discussed previously, all HIV-infected mothers should be counseled on infant feeding. Women with HIV present a risk of transmission through breastmilk and premastication of infant food. Given this concern, it is recommended that women infected with HIV do not breastfeed, despite viral load counts, especially if living in the United States, where there is access to formula, which is a safe and healthy alternative to breastmilk.[19]

FUTURE CONSIDERATIONS

Overall pregnancy is a unique time in a woman's life and is only compounded by a diagnosis of HIV infection. Large strides have been made in the reduction of HIV perinatal transmission with the ART options available for these patients. More research is still needed, however, to create successful and safe options for these women and children. Educating both clinicians and patients should be continued. Education and discussions of management and options should be reviewed, ideally prior to pregnancy. Clinicians and patients are urged to participate in the Antiretroviral Pregnancy Registry reporting (http://www.APRegistry.com).[14] Ideally this registry's data will provide the needed research for a more promising future for these patients and their children.

REFERENCES

1. Centers for Disease Control and Prevention. HIV Basics. Available at: https://www.cdc.gov/hiv/basics/statistics.html. Accessed September 23, 2017.
2. Martin J, Hamilton B, Osterman M, et al. Births: final data for 2015. Natl Vital Stat Rep 2017;66(1):1–70. Available at: https://www.cdc.gov/nchs/data/nvsr/nvsr66/nvsr66_01.pdf.
3. Centers for Disease Control and Prevention. HIV among pregnant women, infants, and children. Available at: https://www.cdc.gov/hiv/group/gender/pregnantwomen/index.html. Accessed September 23, 2017.
4. Centers for Disease Control and Prevention. Monitoring selected national HIV prevention and care objectives by using HIV surveillance data—United States and 6 dependent areas, 2014. HIV Surveillance Supplemental Report 2016; 21(4). Available at: https://www.cdc.gov/hiv/library/reports/surveillance/. Accessed September 23, 2017.
5. HIV among pregnant women, infants, and children. CDC.gov. 2017. Available at: https://www.cdc.gov/hiv/group/gender/pregnantwomen/index.html. Accessed November 11, 2017.
6. The HIV Life Cycle. Understanding HIV/AIDS. 2017. Available at: https://aidsinfo.nih.gov/understanding-hiv-aids/fact-sheets/19/73/the-hiv-life-cycle. Accessed November 11, 2017.
7. Panel on treatment of HIV-infected pregnant women and prevention of perinatal transmission. Recommendations for use of antiretroviral drugs in pregnant HIV-1-infected women for maternal health and interventions to reduce perinatal HIV transmission in the United States. Available at: https://aidsinfo.nih.gov/contentfiles/lvguidelines/PerinatalGL.pdf. Accessed September 25, 2017. p. C1–5.
8. Panel on treatment of HIV-infected pregnant women and prevention of perinatal transmission. Recommendations for use of antiretroviral drugs in pregnant HIV-1-infected women for maternal health and interventions to reduce perinatal

HIV transmission in the United States. 2017. Available at https://aidsinfo.nih.gov/contentfiles/lvguidelines/PerinatalGL.pdf. Accessed November 24, 2017. p. C41–83.

9. Safety and dosing of antiretroviral medications in pregnancy. UpToDate.com. 2017. Available at: https://www.uptodate.com/contents/safety-and-dosing-of-antiretroviral-medications-in-pregnancy?source=see_link&sectionName=Tenofovir&anchor=H44#H1. Accessed November 24, 2017.

10. Antiretroviral and intrapartum management of pregnant HIV-infected women and their infants in resource-rich settings. UpToDate.com. 2017. Available at: https://www.uptodate.com/contents/antiretroviral-and-intrapartum-management-of-pregnant-hiv-infected-women-and-their-infants-in-resource-rich-settings?source=search_result&search=Antiretroviral%20and%20intrapartum&selectedTitle=1~150. Accessed November 24, 2017.

11. Overview of antiretroviral agents used to treat HIV. UpToDate.com. 2017. Available at: https://www.uptodate.com/contents/overview-of-antiretroviral-agents-used-to-treat-hiv?source=search_result&search=hiv%20treatment%20adult&selectedTitle=3~150#H14340701. Accessed November 24, 2017.

12. Panel on treatment of HIV-infected pregnant women and prevention of perinatal transmission. Recommendations for use of antiretroviral drugs in pregnant HIV-1-infected women for maternal health and interventions to reduce perinatal HIV transmission in the United States. Available at: https://aidsinfo.nih.gov/contentfiles/lvguidelines/PerinatalGL.pdf. Accessed September 23, 2017. p. C11–2.

13. Panel on treatment of HIV-infected pregnant women and prevention of perinatal transmission. Recommendations for use of antiretroviral drugs in pregnant HIV-1-infected women for maternal health and interventions to reduce perinatal HIV transmission in the United States. Available at: https://aidsinfo.nih.gov/contentfiles/lvguidelines/PerinatalGL.pdf. Accessed September 23, 2017. p. C20–40.

14. Panel on treatment of HIV-infected pregnant women and prevention of perinatal transmission. Recommendations for use of antiretroviral drugs in pregnant HIV-1-infected women for maternal health and interventions to reduce perinatal HIV transmission in the United States. Available at: https://aidsinfo.nih.gov/contentfiles/lvguidelines/PerinatalGL.pdf. Accessed September 25, 2017. p. C6–10.

15. Prenatal evaluation of the HIV-infected woman in resource-rich settings. UpToDate.com. 2017. Available at: https://www.uptodate.com/contents/prenatal-evaluation-of-the-hiv-infected-woman-in-resource-rich-settings?source=see_link#H10063311. Accessed November 11, 2017.

16. Briggs GG, Freeman RK, Yaffe SJ. Drugs in pregnancy and lactation. 10th edition. Philadelphia: Wolters Kluwer/Lippincott Williams & Wilkins Health; 2014.

17. Panel on treatment of HIV-infected pregnant women and prevention of perinatal transmission. Recommendations for use of antiretroviral drugs in pregnant HIV-1-infected women for maternal health and interventions to reduce perinatal HIV transmission in the United States. 2017. Available at: https://aidsinfo.nih.gov/contentfiles/lvguidelines/PerinatalGL.pdf. Accessed November 24, 2017. p. D1–14.

18. Panel on treatment of HIV-infected pregnant women and prevention of perinatal transmission. Recommendations for use of antiretroviral drugs in pregnant HIV-1-infected women for maternal health and interventions to reduce perinatal

HIV transmission in the United States. 2017. Available at: https://aidsinfo.nih.gov/contentfiles/lvguidelines/PerinatalGL.pdf. Accessed November 24, 2017. p. E1–43.

19. Prevention of HIV transmission during breastfeeding in resource limited settings. UpToDate.com. 2017. Available at: https://www.uptodate.com/contents/prevention-of-hiv-transmission-during-breastfeeding-in-resource-limited-settings?source=search_result&search=hiv%20breastfeeding&selectedTitle=1 ~ 150. Accessed November 24, 2017.

Challenging Vaginas
Case Studies in Recognizing and Treating Vulvovaginitis

Linda Burdette, PA-C, MPAS

KEYWORDS

- Bacterial vaginosis • Vulvovaginal candidiasis • Trichomoniasis
- Vulvovaginal atrophy • Desquamative inflammatory vaginitis

INTRODUCTION

Seventy percent of episodes of vaginitis in premenopausal women are caused by bacterial vaginosis, vulvovaginal candidiasis, and/or trichomoniasis. As our population ages and fewer women are using systemic hormone therapy, we see increasing numbers of vulvovaginal atrophy, making postmenopausal atrophy the most common cause of vulvovaginal discomfort. This article reviews cases that demonstrate the common causes and treatments of vulvovaginitis, the treatment for persistent cases, and the diagnosis and treatment of the less common causes.

CASE 1

Brenda is a 26-year-old sexually active woman who presents with complaints of an increased discharge with a strong odor, especially after her periods and after intercourse. She has no pain with intercourse, periods are monthly, and she is using oral contraceptives to prevent pregnancy. Pelvic examination shows no vulvar or vaginal irritation but there is an increased whitish/gray, homogeneous discharge that clings to the walls and feels slimy during sampling. She has no pain with the examination. You notice a fishy odor to the discharge and when you add KOH to one of the wet mount slides, the odor is even more noticeable (positive whiff or amine test). A pH test of the vaginal secretions is greater than 4.5 and when you look at a wet mount slide under the microscope, there are copious clue cells and few long rods of lactobacilli (a drop of Sedi-Stain, marketed for urine staining, makes the clue cells as obvious as seen in **Fig. 1**).

You make the diagnosis of bacterial vaginosis (BV) and treat her with metronidazole, either oral or vaginal. Brenda returns in 3 months because her symptoms resolved with initial treatment, but are now back.

The author has no commercial or financial conflicts of interest to disclose.
Premier Women's Health of Yakima, 6101 Summitview Avenue, Suite 210, Yakima, WA 98908, USA
E-mail address: lindaburdette@gmail.com

Physician Assist Clin 3 (2018) 411–421
https://doi.org/10.1016/j.cpha.2018.02.009   physicianassistant.theclinics.com
2405-7991/18/© 2018 Elsevier Inc. All rights reserved.

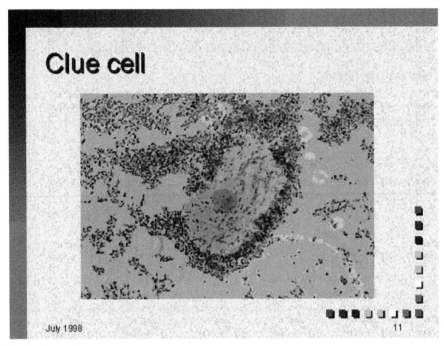

Fig. 1. Clue cell.

Case 1 Discussion

BV is the most prevalent cause of symptomatic vaginal discharge in the United States,[1] and has been associated with complications including preterm delivery of infants, pelvic inflammatory disease, urinary tract infections, and acquisition/transmission of sexually transmitted diseases (STDs), including human immunodeficiency virus (HIV).[2–4] It is marked by a lack of normal hydrogen peroxide–producing lactobacilli and overgrowth of bacteria such as *Gardnerella vaginalis*, *Mycoplasma hominis*, *Atopobium vaginae*, and many other anaerobes. Douching, menstrual flow, and intercourse all provide an environment that is friendlier to this polymicrobial infection. Diagnoses are made clinically with findings of at least 3 of 4 Amsel criteria: homogeneous white/gray discharge that smoothly coats the vaginal walls, vaginal pH >4.5, a positive amine (whiff) test, and more than 20% of the epithelial cells being clue cells. Culture has no role in the diagnosis of BV because *G. vaginalis* is detected more than half of the time in healthy, asymptomatic women.

Treatments for BV approved by the Centers for Disease Control and Prevention (CDC) include the following[5]:

- Metronidazole 500 mg by mouth twice a day × 7 days
- Metronidazole 0.75% gel, 1 full applicator intravaginally daily for 5 days
  - Not to be used during the first 13 weeks of pregnancy
- Clindamycin 2% cream, 1 full applicator vaginally daily for 7 days
- A newly approved medication, as of September 2017, is Secnidazole 2 g granule, an oral, single-dose treatment
- Alternative therapy includes Tinidazole 2 g by mouth daily for 2 days, or
- Tinidazole 1 g by mouth daily for 5 days

- Clindamycin 300 mg by mouth twice a day for 7 days
- Clindamycin ovules 100 g intravaginally at bedtime × 3 nights

Metronidazole is preferred over clindamycin because it is more sparing of lactobacilli,[6] but clindamycin is preferred in cases of allergy or intolerance to metronidazole or tinidazole. Generally, topical therapy is more expensive than generic oral metronidazole, although the latter may be associated with significant gastrointestinal symptoms. Alcohol needs to be avoided for 24 hours after metronidazole use (both oral and topical) and 72 hours after tinidazole use to reduce the possibility of a disulfiramlike reaction (severe nausea and vomiting). Women should be advised to refrain from sexual activity or use condoms consistently and correctly during the treatment regimen.[5]

Recurrent BV occurs commonly within a year of treatment, but the actual number varies with the treatment regimen and many cofactors.[7] Risk factors include having a history of BV, having a regular sex partner, having a female sex partner, and having a low vitamin D level.[7] Protective effects include the use of hormonal contraception. Recent studies have shown that 90% of women with BV have a complex polymicrobial biofilm seen on electron microscopy.[8] Biofilm is slime produced by bacteria that coats surfaces and within which bacteria hide from and are protected from the effects of antibiotics. Antibiotics reduce the bacteria load but do not eliminate it. There is an ongoing debate on sexual transmission, as there can be transmission between female partners, similar flora can be found in male partners of women with BV, and G vaginalis–dominant biofilm has been found in men.[8] However, BV is not considered an STD and in heterosexual couples, randomized studies of partner treatment have failed to show a decrease in the risk of recurrence.[8]

Options for recurrent BV treatment include higher doses and longer courses of the same medications used for initial therapy. They lower the long-term recurrence rates but do not eliminate them, and include the following:

- 10 days of vaginal metronidazole gel 5 g daily and then metronidazole gel twice a week for 4 to 6 months.[6,9] It was noted that secondary vaginal candidiasis occurred more commonly in the treatment group than the placebo control group.
- Oral metronidazole or tinidazole 500 mg by mouth twice a day for 7 days followed by 21 days of boric acid suppositories used vaginally and then metronidazole gel twice weekly for 4 months.[9,10] Ideally, metronidazole gel is continued for 1 to 2 months after normalization of pH.[10] Boric acid suppositories can be made by the patient using the largest empty capsules available at "health food stores"; then she fills them with over-the-counter (OTC) boric acid granules (600 mg per capsule); or, she can order them prefilled online.
- Monthly 2-g single dose of oral metronidazole coadministered with 100 to 200 mg of oral fluconazole,[9] as secondary vaginal candidiasis can occur in metronidazole-treated women.[6]
- Clindamycin 300 mg by mouth twice a day × 7 days, which would need to be stopped if diarrhea starts.[5]
- Routine testing of the partner is not recommended at this point. Most researchers who suspect the onset of BV is related to sexual activity recommend condom use, but a few are treating the partners with oral metronidazole.[11] BV may be transmitted between female sexual partners.[5]
- Oral and vaginal probiotics also are being evaluated. In the study by Ya and colleagues,[12] vaginal preparations (with each capsule containing 8 billion units *Lactobacillus rhamnosus, Lactobacillus acidophilus*, and *Streptococcus thermophiles*), being used 7 days on, 7 days off, 7 on, showed lower recurrence rates than placebo at 2-month and 11-month follow-up. Dr Hillary Liss, MD, MPH, in

a recent University of Washington STD Prevention Training advised that most probiotic preparations are of bovine origin and will not benefit the vagina, the exception being *Lactobacillus crispatus* which might have potential as a vaginal probiotic suppository.[9,11]

- Advise your patients to consider condom use following treatment to allow the vaginal ecosystem time to heal. Clean sex toys after each use. Avoid douching, spermatocides, and multiple sexual partners. Make sure her 25-hydroxyvitamin D serum level is adequate; studies are mixed on the effectiveness of this helping with BV prevention however.

Key Points
- Standard therapy for BV is effective but recurrence rate is very high.
- Higher doses and longer courses of treatment lower long-term recurrence rates.

CASE 2

Carmen is a 60-year-old woman who presents with vulvar itching and burning for the past 2 months. It started after a course of antibiotics for a cellulitis on her leg. She is obese and diabetic, admitting to poor glucose control. She has tried one OTC product for yeast that made her burn even more. She also used one "leftover" fluconazole pill early in the course of her symptoms with moderate, but temporary relief. Pelvic examination shows vulvar obesity with symmetric erythematous rash on the labia majora extending laterally to the groin folds and inferiorly to the gluteal crease. The labia minora are very tender and friable, appearing almost white on the medial aspect and erythematous laterally. Fissuring is seen at the posterior fourchette. The vagina is pale pink and there is a small amount of clear discharge. If the diagnosis is in question, the vagina and vulva can be swabbed for Candida DNA testing (polymerase chain reaction [PCR]) to confirm the presence and type of Candida. If you test the pH, it is <4.7, and the wet mount might or might not show budding yeast.

Without waiting for the PCR results, you make the preliminary diagnosis of vulvovaginal candidiasis based on her history and physical findings, and assume the offending agent is most likely *Candida albicans*. Because of the length of time she has had the symptoms and her diabetes history, you determine this is a complicated vulvovaginal candidiasis and anticipate a lengthier course of treatment will be necessary, starting her on oral fluconazole 150 mg by mouth every 3 days for 3 doses and then weekly[5] until you recheck her in 2 to 4 weeks. Alternatively, 100-mg or 200-mg fluconazole doses can be used if those doses are accepted better by her insurance.

Case 2 Discussion

Vulvovaginal candidiasis is a common infection affecting most (70%–75%) women at least once during their reproductive years, and 40% to 50% of women more than once.[13] Antimicrobials are thought to predispose a patient to Candida by reducing the number of protective resident vaginal bacteria. The primary symptom is vulvar pruritus; however, burning, soreness, and irritation also are common. Women will often present with vulvar edema, fissures, and excoriations secondary to scratching. Secondary bacterial cellulitis can occur. Patients may complain of burning with urination or dyspareunia. The classic vaginal discharge is thick, white, and clumpy, but the infection can be present without this discharge appearance. Erythematous tissues may be seen in the vagina, vestibule, labia minora, labia majora, or not at all. Wet mount with either saline or KOH preparation may show budding yeast and hyphae. The pH will be less than 4.5. The primary culprit is *C albicans*, found in up to 90% of all cases. Recurrent vulvovaginal candidiasis, presenting with itching, burning, and fissuring, should be differentiated from herpes simplex, which may present similarly. Vulvar cellulitis should be considered if there is a swollen, beefy-red appearance and the patient presents with aching pain, tenderness, chills, fever, or lymphadenopathy.[14]

All OTC imidazoles (eg, butoconazole, clotrimazole, miconazole) and prescription single-dose oral fluconazole have similar efficacy for C albicans and are good choices for uncomplicated infections. Remind patients that the 1-day, 3-day, and 7-day courses of topical medications may all take 7 days for complete resolution of her symptoms. The Guidelines from the Centers for Disease Control and Prevention is a good resource on the lengthy list of first-line OTC therapies for vulvovaginal candidiasis.[5] Recurrent or more severe infections may be treated with an extended 14-day course of the topical medications, and pregnant patients are best treated with a 7-day topical course.[5]

Complicated vulvovaginal candidiasis is based on having any of the following[5]:

- Four or more episodes in a year
- Severe symptoms or findings
- Suspected or proven non-albican Candida infection
- Women with diabetes
- Severe medical illness
- Immunosuppression
- Other vulvovaginal conditions
- Pregnancy

PRC results will identify the causative organism; if her infection is not caused by the most common C albicans, consider the following:

- With Candida glabrata (which occurs in 8% of cases) there will be 50% improvement with the "azoles"; Candida parapsilosis will show 40% improvement.[15]
- C glabrata may respond to topical Gentian Violet treatment and it is easy to have an inexpensive bottle in each examination room to apply with a small applicator to affected tissue at the conclusion of your examination.[16]
- C glabrata may respond to treatment with vaginal boric acid, 600 mg, daily in gelatin capsule for 14 days in capsules, as discussed earlier.[15]
- C glabrata may respond to flucytosine compounded into 15.5% vaginal cream, 5 g daily for 14 days, with or without amphotericin B 50-mg suppositories given nightly.[17]

Persistent vulvovaginal candidiasis may be related to antimicrobial resistance and to biofilm production[18] (similar to that seen in BV). Maintenance fluconazole may be indicated for complicated candidiasis by continuing the weekly dose of fluconazole for up to 6 months.[19] This is also a good time to encourage your patient to work on weight loss and better control of her diabetes if those are coexisting factors.

CASE 2 (CONTINUED)

On the follow-up examination, Carmen's PCR results showed she had a C albicans infection and the erythematous appearance of the labia majora has improved. What remains though, and still causes her intense itching, are the changes in the labia minora. Here you note that the medial aspect looks like "cigarette paper" in color and thickness and she still has the fissuring at the posterior fourchette. This is consistent with lichen sclerosus (LS), and you realize this patient has had a mixture of etiologies causing her distress.

Case 2 Discussion (Continued)

LS (previously known as LS&A for lichen sclerosus et atrophicus) (**Fig. 2**), a chronic disorder of the skin, is characterized by itching, depigmentation (hypopigmentation) frequently in an hourglass pattern, and loss of mucocutaneous markings (labial resorption).

Symptoms may progress to submucosal hemorrhage, fissuring, ulcerations, burying of the clitoris, and even complete fusion of the labia minora.[14] The vagina is typically spared. The etiology is uncertain, but an autoimmune process or genetic link is likely, and it is much more common in hypoestrogen states of postmenopause and occasionally prepubertal girls.

The vulva is steroid-resistant so an ultrapotent steroid is necessary to affect change. Ointments are preferred to creams or lotions that can be drying and irritating. Clobetasol propionate 0.05% ointment applied daily for 4 weeks is recommended.[20] As LS has a lifetime risk of development of vulvar squamous cell carcinoma,[14] a biopsy should be taken either before treatment or after a month of treatment if your patient has not had reasonable resolution of her symptoms and mucocutaneous ulcerations or atypical thickening is identified. There is some controversy regarding the need for maintenance therapy, with some experts recommending treatment only of flares and others recommending twice-weekly application of ultrapotent or

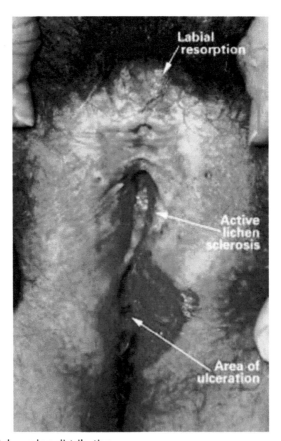

Fig. 2. Vulvar LS: hourglass distribution.

moderate-strength steroid.[21] Continued monitoring is advised at least once a year when you are satisfied with the patient's response.

Key Points
- Complicated vulvovaginal candidiasis requires extended treatment
- Vulvovaginitis may have multiple etiologies at the same time
- If LS does not respond to ultrapotency steroids, a biopsy should be performed to rule out vulvar carcinoma

CASE 3

Terri is a 22-year-old who is complaining of increased greenish vaginal discharge and pain with intercourse and urination. She complains that her vagina feels sore and itchy. She is sexually active and has been with 2 different men in the past 3 months. She has no increased frequency of urination or nocturia. She uses an intrauterine device for contraception and prefers not using condoms. Her examination shows generalized erythema to the vaginal walls with a purulent, bubbly discharge. No punctate hemorrhages are seen. During the examination you obtain a vaginal specimen for gonorrhea and chlamydia testing, and you draw a serology specimen for HIV and syphilis testing. Microscopy confirms motile trichomonads and an abundance of white blood cells. Making a diagnosis of trichomonas vaginalis, there are 3 CDC treatment recommendation options:

- Metronidazole, 2 g by mouth in a single dose
- Tinidazole 2 g by mouth in a single dose
- Metronidazole 500 mg by mouth twice a day for 7 days[5]

You treat her with the single dose of metronidazole, hoping for the best compliance, recommend treatment or write prescriptions for her sexual partners, explain the concept of sexually transmitted infections, and inform her that she should not have intercourse with either of her partners until they have all completed treatment. You advise the use of condoms for all sexual encounters. You also advise her that alcohol should be avoided during metronidazole use and for 24 hours after.

Case 3 Discussion

Trichomoniasis is the first STD presented in this article. An elevated vaginal pH is seen but the diagnosis relies on visualization of motile trichomonads on saline microscopy. A wet mount has a sensitivity of 55% to 60% in diagnosing trichomoniasis.[22] A point-of-care test for trichomonas antigen, the OSOM Trichomonas Rapid Antigen test, has a sensitivity of 88.3% and specificity of 98.8%, and is an alternative for testing, especially if microscopy is not available.[23] Aptima PCR testing can be sent to the laboratory as a third alternative, with 100% sensitivity and 98.2% specificity listed in its performance data. The classic "strawberry cervix" caused by punctate hemorrhages is uncommonly seen on the visual component of the examination.

Terri returns in 3 weeks because her symptoms have improved but are not completely resolved. Her partners took the medication and she has used condoms since treatment. Microscopy again confirms motile trichomonads. Persistent cases occur because of noncompliance, reinfection, or metronidazole resistance, which is estimated between 1.7% and 10.0%.[24] Recommended metronidazole regimens have resulted in cure rates of approximately 84% to 98%, and the recommended tinidazole regimen has resulted in cure rates of approximately 92% to 100%.[5] Tinidazole is more effective and has fewer gastrointestinal side effects, but it is more expensive[5] and may be more difficult to obtain insurance approval. Secondary to the high cost of tinidazole, you treat her the second time with a longer course of metronidazole,

500 mg by mouth twice a day for 7 days.[5] You advise her not to have intercourse until you recheck her wet mount following treatment. If the second treatment fails, consider one of the following:

- Metronidazole or tinidazole 2 g by mouth for 7 days[5]
- Metronidazole or tinidazole 500 mg by mouth 4 times daily for 14 days[25]
- Metronidazole 500 mg by mouth twice a day for 7 days, followed by 2 g by mouth daily for an additional 5 days[25]
- Tinidazole 1 g by mouth 2 to 3 times a day along with 500 mg vaginally for 14 days[25]
- Sending the resistant isolate to a reference laboratory that can perform susceptibility testing should be considered if the above treatments are not successful.

Key points
- Persistent trichomoniasis occurs because of noncompliance, reinfection, or metronidazole resistance
- Higher dose and longer interval treatment options are available

CASE 4

Anna, a 62-year-old woman, presents with symptoms of vaginal dryness, occasional itching and burning, and painful intercourse. She has been menopausal for 10 years; she took systemic hormone therapy (HT) for 5 years and then was advised to stop HT by her health care provider. She uses a water-based lubricant for intercourse. Physical examination shows pale vulvar tissues that have lost their fullness; the vaginal tissues are pale, thin, and dry, being very sensitive to insertion and opening of the speculum. Further examination shows an elevated vaginal pH (6.0–7.5) and the presence of parabasal or intermediate cells on microscopy. An amine test is negative. Your diagnosis is postmenopausal vulvovaginal atrophy (VVA) or genitourinary syndrome of menopause.

Up to 50% of all postmenopausal women will experience vulvovaginal irritation, soreness and dryness, lower urinary tract symptoms, and dyspareunia.[26] Perimenopausal women can also experience vulvar irritation and dryness. Even with the use of systemic HT, some women will experience symptoms of atrophy as the vulvovaginal tissues are the most estrogen-dependent tissues in the body. Besides pallor of tissues, loss of rugal folds, petechiae or frank bleeding, loss of elasticity, narrowing of the introitus and shortening of the vagina can be seen. The thinning of the tissues will sometimes present with a hyperemic appearance instead of pallor. Minimal discharge is typical of atrophy, but in some advanced cases a dark yellow or brown discharge will be visualized and maybe even noticed by the patient.

First-line therapy is usually using personal lubricants with intercourse, with silicone-based lubricants decreasing friction more than water-based lubricants. Nonhormonal OTC vaginal moisturizers (such as Replens), inserted every 2 to 3 days, also may be helpful as well as increased sexual intercourse. For more advanced cases, systemic estrogen or low-dose topical vaginal estrogen is the treatment of choice. For this patient, topical estrogen would be appropriate. Vaginal estradiol is available as a cream, suppository, or a 3-month ring. Vaginal conjugated equine estrogen is also available as a cream, as well as a daily oral selective estrogen receptor modulator, ospemifene. Recently a new product, a once-daily vaginal insert, has received approval by the Food and Drug Administration (FDA) for dyspareunia due to menopause; prasterone is the active ingredient, which is also known as DHEA. Cost and convenience will determine which product is best for your patient; the estradiol suppository option is the only one currently available as a generic.

In women with a current or prior history of breast cancer, data do not show an increased risk of cancer recurrence with the use of vaginal estrogen to relieve urogenital symptoms.[27] Concerns remain, however, about recurrence risk with use of vaginal estrogen in women with breast cancer who use aromatase inhibitors,[28] and consultation with the patient's oncologist is advised. Women on aromatase inhibitors who experience urogenital symptoms refractory to nonhormonal approaches may benefit from the short-term use of estrogen with tamoxifen to improve symptoms, followed by a return to normal aromatase inhibitor therapy for the duration of the treatment course.[29] Graduated vaginal dilators may be helpful to treat or prevent introital narrowing, and are cheaper for patients to order online than through a medical equipment supplier.

Fractional carbon dioxide laser treatment for vaginal atrophy is being advertised and used recently. The position statement of the American College of Obstetricians and Gynecologists (ACOG) of May 2016 states, "this technology is, in fact, neither approved nor cleared by the FDA for the specific indication of treating vulvovaginal atrophy."[30] Preliminary observational data have shown some potential benefits with the use of this technology in treating patients with VVA; however, these trials do not evaluate the use of concomitant treatments, and the follow-up was only for 12 weeks. ACOG advises providing accurate and current information to patients for them to be fully engaged in the informed decision-making process.[30]

Key points
- 50% of postmenopausal women will experience the side effects of VVA
- Estrogen therapy has been the standard of care with new treatment options becoming recently available

LESS COMMON CAUSES

Almost any condition that can occur on the skin can occur on the vulva. Remember to take a thorough history regarding skin conditions existing on other parts of the body, such as atopic dermatitis/eczema, seborrheic dermatitis, and psoriasis, as they may also exist on vulvar tissues. Take a history of any products that have been used on the urogenital area. Anti-itch/numbing creams and fabric softeners frequently can cause contact dermatitis, or in other words, more itching. This may lead to lichen simplex, also known as chronic lichenified dermatitis with the appearance of thickened, leathery skin. Contact allergens can even include medications that have been prescribed. Aggressive cleansing, medicated wipes, and douching strip normal protections from the vulva and vagina, and should be avoided. Forgotten tampons and condoms are some of the more common foreign bodies that can be found in the vagina causing abnormal discharge or odor.

Of the rarer forms of vaginitis, desquamative inflammatory vaginitis (DIV) should be remembered. This is a chronic clinical syndrome of unknown etiology, generally occurring in perimenopausal or postmenopausal women, with symptoms of burning, dyspareunia, and abnormal yellow or green discharge. Some have argued that DIV may represent a vaginal expression of erosive lichen planus.[31] Examination reveals purulent discharge with varying amount of vestibular and/or vaginal erythema. The pH is elevated and the amine test is negative. Microscopy reveals large amounts of white blood cells and parabasal cells. This condition clinically may be mistaken for trichomoniasis but no motile trichomonads are present on microscopy or cultures. Treatment options include the following:

- A 14-day course with 2% clindamycin vaginal cream often will achieve a cure; however, relapse after therapy is fairly common[32]

- The University of Washington Department of Gynecology treatment regimen is much longer. A 21-day course with using an applicator of 2% clindamycin cream nightly is followed by a 14-day course of the clindamycin cream every other day. Then for 28 days, the patient has 4-day cycles of clindamycin cream, nothing, Anusol HC (hydrocortisone) rectal suppositories in the vagina, nothing; this cycle is repeated 7 times. Personal experience has shown excellent results with infrequent relapses IF the patient starts and continues vaginal estrogen as soon as this regimen has been completed.

A referral for any challenging vagina or vulvar presentation is sometimes necessary. Interestingly, a survey of 200 patients at a tertiary vaginitis center with symptoms lasting more than a year showed 21% were caused by contact dermatitis, 21% by recurrent vulvovaginal candidiasis, 15% by atrophic vaginitis, and 13% by localized provoked vestibulodynia; 9% were physiologic discharge; and 18% had 2 or more concurrent diagnoses.[33] And as a word of caution, consider a vulvar biopsy, particularly if you are dealing with hyperpigmented or exophytic lesions, lesions with changes in vascular patterns, or unresolving lesions, to rule out carcinoma.[34]

REFERENCES

1. Fleury FJ. Adult vaginitis. Clin Obstet Gynecol 1981;24:407–38.
2. Eschenbach DA. Bacterial vaginosis and anaerobes in obstetric-gynecologic infection. Clin Infect Dis 1993;16:S282–7.
3. Hillier S. The vaginal microbial ecosystem and resistance to HIV. AIDS Res Hum Retroviruses 1998;14:S17–21.
4. Martin HL, Richardson BA, Nyange PM, et al. Vaginal lactobacilli, microbial flora, and risk of human immunodeficiency virus type 1 and sexually transmitted disease acquisition. J Infect Dis 1999;180:1863–8.
5. CDC 2015 Sexually Transmitted Disease Treatment Guidelines. Available at: https://www.cdc.gov/std/tg2015/bv.htm. Accessed March 22, 2018.
6. Sobel JD, Faro S, Force RW, et al. Suppressive antibacterial therapy. Am J Obstet Gynecol 2006;194:1283–9.
7. Bradshaw CS, Morton AN, Hocking J, et al. High recurrence rates of bacterial vaginosis over the course of 12 months after oral metronidazole therapy and factors associated with recurrence. J Infect Dis 2006;193:1478–86.
8. Verstraelen H, Swidsinski A. The biofilm in BV. Curr Opin Infect Dis 2013;26:86–9.
9. Liss H. Yakima (WA): University of Washington STD Prevention Training Center; 2017.
10. Reichman O, Akins R, Sobel JD. Boric acid addition to suppressive antimicrobial therapy for recurrent bacterial vaginosis. Sex Transm Dis 2009;36:732–4.
11. Wilson J. Managing recurrent bacterial vaginosis. BMJ Journals 2004;80(1). https://doi.org/10.1136/sti.2002.002733.
12. Ya W, Reifer C, Miller LE. Efficacy of vaginal probiotics capsules for recurrent bacterial vaginosis. Am J Obstet Gynecol 2010;203(2):120.e1-6.
13. Sobel JD. Epidemiology and pathogenesis of recurrent vulvovaginal candidiasis. Am J Obstet Gynecol 1985;152:924–35.
14. Haque Hussain S, Sterling J. Skin diseases affecting the vulva. Obstetrics, Gynaecology and Reproductive Medicine 2014.
15. Sobel JD, Chaim W, Nagappan V, et al. Treatment of vaginitis caused by *C glabrata*: use of topical boric acid and flucytosine. Am J Obstet Gynecol 2003;189: 1297–300.

16. Iavazzo C, Gkegkes ID, Zarkada IM, et al. Boric acid for recurrent vulvovaginal candidiasis: the clinical evidence. J Womens Health 2011;20(8):1245–55.
17. Phillips AF. Treatment of non-albicans Candida vag with amphotericin B vaginal supp. Am J Obstet Gynecol 2005;192:2009–12.
18. Paiva LC, Vidigal VG, Donatti L, et al. Assessment of in vitro biofilm formation by Candida isolates from vulvovaginal candidiasis and ultrastructural characteristics. Micron 2012;43(2–3):497–502.
19. Sobel JD, Wiesenfield HC, Martens M, et al. Maintenance fluconazole therapy for recurrent vulvovaginal candidiasis. N Engl J Med 2004;351:876–83.
20. Neill SM, Tatnall FM, Cox NH, British Association of Dermatologists. Guidelines for the management of lichen sclerosus. Br J Dermatol 2002;147:640–9.
21. Renaud-Vilmer C, Cavelier-Balloy B, Porcher R, et al. Vulvar lichen sclerosus: effect of long-term topical application of a potent steroid on the course of the disease. Arch Dermatol 2004;140:709–12.
22. Krieger JN, Tam MR, Stevens CE, et al. Diagnosis of trichomoniasis. Comparison of conventional wet-mount examination with cytologic studies, cultures, and monoclonal antibody staining of direct specimens. JAMA 1988;259:1223–7.
23. Huppert JS, Batteiger BE, Braslins P, et al. Use of an immunochromoatographic assay for rapid detection of trichomonas vaginalis in vaginal specimens. J Clin Microbiol 2005;43:684–7.
24. Krashin JW, Koumans EH, Bradshaw-Sydnor AC, et al. Trich vag prevalence, incidence, risk factors and antibiotic-resistance in an adolescent population. Sex Transm Dis 2009;37:440–4.
25. Sobel JD, Nyirjesy P, Brown W. Tinidazole therapy for metronidazole-resistant vaginal trichomoniasis. Clin Infect Dis 2001;33:1341–6.
26. Greendale GA, Judd HL. The menopause: health implication and clinical management. J Am Geriatr Soc 1993;41:426–36.
27. Ponzone R, Biglia N, Jacomuzzi ME. Vaginal oestrogen therapy after breast cancer; is it safe? Eur J Cancer 2005;41:2673–81.
28. Trinkaus M, Chin S, Wolfman W. Should urogenital atrophy in breast cancer survivors be treated with topical estrogens? Oncologist 2008;13:222–31.
29. Kendall A, Dowsett M, Folkerd E, et al. Caution: vaginal estradiol appears to be contraindicated in postmenopausal women on adjuvant aromatase inhibitors. Ann Oncol 2006;17:584–7.
30. American College of Obstetricians and Gynecologists. Fractional laser treatment of vulvovaginal atrophy and U.S. Food and Drug Administration Clearance Position Statement. 2016. Available at: https://www.acog.org/Clinical-Guidance-and-Publications/Position-Statements/Fractional-Laser-Treatment-of-Vulvovaginal-Atrophy-and-US-Food-and-Drug-Administration-Clearance. Accessed March 22, 2018.
31. Edwards L, Friedrich DF Jr. Desquamative vaginitis: lichen planus in disguise. Obstet Gynecol 1988;71:8332–6.
32. Sobel JD. Desquamative inflammatory vaginitis: a new subgroup of purulent vaginitis responsive to topical 2% clindamycin therapy. Am J Obstet Gynecol 1994; 171:1214–20.
33. Nyirjesy P, Peyton C, Weitz MV, et al. Causes of chronic vaginitis: analysis of a prospective database of affected women. Obstet Gynecol 2006;108:1185–91.
34. Jones RW, Joura EA. Analyzing prior clinical events at presentation in 102 women with vulvar carcinoma. Evidence of diagnostic delays. J Reprod Med 1999;44: 766–8.

A Review of Infertility for the Primary Care Provider

Sarah Lindahl, PA-C

KEYWORDS

- Infertility • Female infertility • Male infertility • Subfertility
- Hypothalamic dysfunction • Diminished ovarian reserve • Fecundability
- Preimplantation genetic screening

KEY POINTS

- Difficulty becoming pregnant is a common phenomenon seen in health care, but it is believed that most cases relate to subfertility rather than infertility or sterility.
- Causes of infertility are vast and varied, can relate to both male and female pathology, and are not definitively identified in approximately one-third of couples presenting with inability to become pregnant when they want to.
- The evaluation of infertility should encompass a work-up of both members of a couple, starting with detailed history and physical examination, semen analysis, and serum hormone studies.
- Considerations regarding management of infertility should address the goals of a couple, financial implication and insurance coverage, and potential need for referral to a reproductive endocrinologist and infertility specialist and should start with least invasive measures.

INTRODUCTION

It is estimated that 1 in 8 couples experience infertility. Experience with infertility is often described as isolating, frustrating, and depressing. Physician assistants can help their patients during this difficult time by providing accurate information and helpful emotional support. This article reviews the definitions of infertility, how to conduct and interpret the infertility work-up, and how to assist patients as they navigate through treatments offered by a reproductive specialist.

DEFINING INFERTILITY

This discussion starts by asking the question, What is normal fertility? The study most commonly referenced was data collected from 5574 couples between the years 1946

Disclosure: None.
Sutter East Bay Medical Foundation, 20101 Lake Chabot Road, Floor 3, Castro Valley, CA 94546, USA
E-mail address: shlindobgyn@yahoo.com

Physician Assist Clin 3 (2018) 423–432
https://doi.org/10.1016/j.cpha.2018.02.013   physicianassistant.theclinics.com

to 1956. It was noted that 50% became pregnant after 6 months and 85% were pregnant by the end of 1 year.[1] Although these data was collected more than 70 years ago, other studies with much smaller sample sizes have shown similar results. It was further calculated that fecundability (ability to become pregnant) is 0.25 in the first 3 months of trying to conceive and drops to 0.15 for the next 9 months. These numbers represent the percentage chance of pregnancy for a healthy couple with no reproductive barriers. One of the most inherent challenges to fertility is that human reproduction is inefficient. The woman produces 1 gamete per month and there is a narrow window of time in which fertilization can occur. Although only 1 sperm is needed, men have millions of gametes at their disposal at any time.

Nonetheless, the timeframe of 1 year without conception has been accepted as the point to begin an infertility work-up in women under the age of 35. Accepting that age is an important contributing factor to infertility, it has been suggested that the work-up can take place after 6 months for women older than 35.[2] These timeframes apply to starting the investigation, not establishing a diagnosis of infertility. Some investigators argue that with the exception of a few diagnoses (premature ovarian failure, nonobstructive azoospermia, bilateral tubal occlusion, Asherman syndrome, or severe müllerian abnormalities), most couples seeking fertility evaluation or treatments are really subfertile, meaning they have a decreased potential for conception rather than a complete inability to become pregnant. Yet, for practical purposes, patients define infertility as the inability to be pregnant when they want to be.

ETIOLOGY OF INFERTILITY

Arriving at a definitive diagnosis for infertility or subfertility can be difficult. Sometimes a work-up identifies several factors contributing to a couple's inability to conceive, or it may reveal no explanation at all. A frequently referenced study offers the following breakdown: male factor infertility attributes 26% of the time; the ovary (premature ovarian failure, diminished reserve, polycystic ovarian syndrome [PCOS], or hypothalamic amenorrhea) accounts for 21% of cases; fallopian tube disorders represent 14% of cases, with 6% related to endometriosis; sexual dysfunction may be responsible 6% of the time; cervical stenosis may represent 3% of infertile causes; and approximately 28% of infertile couples do not have an identified causal factor and are labeled as "unexplained."[3]

EVALUATION OF INFERTILITY

It is important to review examples of advice that are not helpful when a patient seeks evaluation and treatment of infertility or subfertility. Many women who struggle with infertility have heard these words from their health care providers: "You're trying too hard; relax and take a vacation!", "You're young, I'm sure everything is fine.", and "I once had a patient who was told she couldn't become pregnant. She tried multiple treatments that didn't work, then she gave up completely and found out she was pregnant." Stress only contributes to infertility through potential hypothalamic dysfunction, menstrual cycle irregularities, and negative affect on sexual performance.[3] Gametes do not have any cognitive powers to be aware if a couple is trying to conceive or are too focused on conception. A tropical location does not enhance fertility and correlation is not causation. Women of various ages can present with infertility and it can be difficult to predict which are affected.

The first step in the evaluation of an infertile couple starts with a detailed history, including history of previous pregnancy and outcomes of those pregnancies, length of time the woman has been actively pursuing pregnancy, and any fertility awareness methods that the woman has been using (menstrual cycle charting, ovulation predictor kits [OPKs], and basal body temperature [BBT] measurements). Obtaining detailed information about a patient's menstrual history can establish if she has regular and predictable cycles or more variable and unpredictable. Characteristics of heavy and painful periods may suggest conditions, such as endometriosis, and patients who describe premenstrual symptoms, such as breast tenderness, bloating, and acne, are likely having ovulatory cycles. Next it is important to ask how often a couple is having intercourse and when. Infrequent or mistimed intercourse is often identified as a couple's failure to conceive. It is well established that the fertile period spans from 5 days before ovulation to 1 day after ovulation, with the highest rates of pregnancy occurring when intercourse takes place daily or every other day and spanning from 2 days before ovulation to the day of ovulation.

It is also important to assess chronic medical conditions, such as hypertension, diabetes, thyroid disease, and other autoimmune disorders, because it is imperative to make sure these disease states are well managed and optimized prior to the start of pregnancy. Discussion and documentation of previous gynecologic diagnoses should be included: ovarian cysts, PCOS, uterine fibroids, hydrosalpinx, sexually transmitted infections, and treatment of pelvic inflammatory disease. Prior surgeries, such as a diagnostic laparoscopy, any ovarian or uterine surgery, salpingectomy for an ectopic pregnancy, or treatments of abnormal Pap smears, should be noted. Any patients with a cancer history should be asked about radiation or chemotherapy treatments because these can affect fertility. Other questions should include asking about personal lifestyle factors, such as occupation, exercise, tobacco, and alcohol and drug use.

Female Evaluation

Evaluation of fertility is divided into the individual components that contribute to pregnancy: ovaries, sperm, fallopian tubes, and uterus. The ovaries are discussed first. The traditional approach has been to measure a follicle-stimulating hormone (FSH) and estradiol (E2) level on day 2 or day 3 of the menstrual cycle. The first limitation with this approach is that it is not assessing the ovarian reserve but rather reveals information about the communication between the hypothalamus/anterior pituitary and the ovaries, which lends some insight into the ovarian reserve. It is an indirect measure, but higher FSH levels indicate a less responsive ovary and suggest a lower ovarian reserve. An expected value is an FSH less than 9.0 mIU/mL, but measuring the E2 level assures the validity of the FSH result. Higher estrogen levels falsely suppress the FSH through the negative feedback loop of the hypothalamic-pituitary-ovarian axis. E2 needs to be less than 80 pg/mL to uphold the FSH value. The other limitation with measuring FSH/E2 levels is that it creates a logistical burden for patients who may have to make another trip to a laboratory, but FSH/E2 levels can vary from month to month, which limits its reliability. More fertility specialists find FSH levels more helpful to predict response to ovarian stimulation than to assess fertility potential.[4]

A more useful tool to assess ovarian reserve is to measure an antimüllerian hormone (AMH) level. AMH is produced by granulosa cells in early antral follicles and the amount present can reflect the depth of the primordial follicle pool. It reaches its highest point in puberty and then declines along the life span and is undetectable by the time a woman reaches menopause. It is consistent within the menstrual cycle and from cycle to cycle. Because it is not influenced by any other feedback mechanism, it can be measured at any time during the cycle or even in a patient who is taking hormonal birth control. A patient who has an AMH value between 2.0 ng/mL and 3.0 ng/mL is considered to have a good ovarian reserve and normal expected fertility. A value less than 1.0 ng/mL is concerning for a decreased (or diminished) ovarian reserve (DOR) and a patient with an AMH less than 0.1 ng/mL has almost no potential for pregnancy with her own eggs. A value greater than 4.0 ng/mL can be suggestive of PCOS in a patient who exhibits other signs and clinical symptoms of PCOS but is not diagnostic on its own.[5]

The other component of evaluating the ovaries is determining not only the supply but also their function in ovulation. The most accurate method of confirming ovulation is with a midluteal phase progesterone level greater than 3.0 ng/mL. This prompts a conversation to make sure a patient knows when her fertile window is occurring. Unfortunately, many textbooks and pamphlets describe a 28-day cycle as the typical menstrual cycle and indicate that ovulation occurs on day 14, which could lead patients to believe that ovulation always occurs on day 14 or perhaps at the midpoint of the cycle. Remember that the reference of a 28-day menstrual cycle is based on an average. Some women have shorter cycles and some have longer cycles. For example, in the absence of a luteal phase defect, a patient with a 26-day cycle ovulates on day 12, whereas a patient with a 32-day cycle ovulates on day 18. It is important to ensure that the app calculates a patient's actual menstrual cycle length to identify that ovulation occurs 14 days before the period begins. Alternatively, women can manually track their cycle length and predict ovulation with use of a traditional calendar.

BBT charting can be a reliable method of confirming ovulation, but it must be done consistently and correctly. Patients need to purchase an oral thermometer but read to 1/100 of a degree to pick up subtle changes not detected by a regular thermometer. The temperature must be recorded first thing at the same time each morning and charted on a graph. A spike and persistent elevation of 0.3°F in the BBT confirms ovulation. A slight dip in the BBT toward the end of the luteal phase suggests the onset of menses, whereas a persistent elevation can be suggestive of an early pregnancy. Although temperature charting may be useful for confirming ovulation, it is not helpful for giving an advance warning on when ovulation may occur.

Patients may ask about using the over-the-counter OPKs. The premise of OPKs is that patients test their urine on a daily basis (between 10:00 AM and 2:00 PM is optimal) and the test strip detects the surge of luteinizing hormone (LH), alerting the woman that ovulation will occur in the next 24 hours to 48 hours. OPKs do not work for all women, however, and both false-positive and false-negative results have been reported. There is a monitor that measures both estrogen and LH levels that may offer more accuracy.

The next component of evaluating the female partner is an assessment of the fallopian tubes and uterus. The hysterosalpingogram (HSG) is the most commonly used imaging study to assess tubal patency and, to some extent, the uterine cavity. After a small catheter is inserted into the cervix, dye is injected into the uterus and its flow is observed under fluoroscopy to determine tubal patency. It should be performed just after the end of the menstrual period but before anticipated ovulation because it may have a therapeutic effect. A review of 12 randomized control trials found that pregnancy rates were higher in subfertile women who had an HSG with oil-soluble media versus women who did not have an HSG with water-soluble media[6] (it is important to know which materials are used at the referring radiology center before advocating a potentially therapeutic effect). As the dye is traveling through the uterus to get to the fallopian tubes, it can help highlight any cavity defects, such as a uterine septum or bicornuate uterus, or any submucosal fibroids. False-negative results are common so a saline sonogram or hysteroscopy should be performed to confirm a cavity defect suggested by the HSG or if any other uterine cavity abnormalities are suspected.

Male Evaluation

The evaluation of the male partner starts with the semen analysis. It is important to be familiar with the services of the local laboratories because not all perform a semen analysis, and some only do a limited evaluation for postvasectomy patients and not a more detailed analysis for infertility. Abstinence from ejaculation 2 days to 7 days prior to collection is recommended. It is also optimal to have the collection (via masturbation) be performed at a laboratory, but it may be obtained and home and transported to the laboratory within 1 hour. Because there can be wide variability of sperm concentrations, it is also helpful to analyze at least 2 samples that were collected with a minimal 1-week interval. The World Health Organization has published reference values for semen analysis based on studies of more than 1900 men who achieved a pregnancy in less than 1 year's time[7]:

Volume—1.5 mL
Sperm concentration—15 million spermatozoa/mL
Total sperm number—39 million per ejaculate
Morphology—4% normal forms
Vitality—58% live
Progressive motility—32%
Total (progressive and nonprogressive) motility—40%

Men with abnormal values benefit from a referral to a urologist or a male fertility specialist before the couple establishes with a reproductive endocrinologist and infertility (REI) specialist. Although REIs are familiar with the causes of male factor infertility, their training and expertise is in women's health rather than evaluation of the male partner. The work-up with a urologist or andrologist should include measuring serum total testosterone, LH, and FSH to assess degrees of hypergonadotropic or hypogonadotropic hypogonadism. These results can also determine any further testing, such as a karyotype to look for Klinefelter syndrome, or other genetic testing for a possible cystic fibrosis gene mutation.[8] A physical examination and ultrasound to identify any varicoceles may determine if a patient has an obstructive (and possibly correctable) versus a nonobstructive azoospermia.

MANAGEMENT OF INFERTILITY

Receiving a recommendation to seek help from a fertility specialist likely feels overwhelming to patients, who may express concern about the expense and invasiveness of infertility treatments, which may not work or may result in a multiple-gestation pregnancy. A provider can help alleviate some of this anxiety by being familiar with the services offered by the fertility specialists in the area. Too often, patients presume that their insurance does not cover anything related to fertility and are prepared to pay for everything out of pocket. Encourage patients to research their benefits and explore their options during open enrollment. Many will be surprised to learn that they have some insurance coverage for diagnostic procedures, medications, or even some treatments. Some states even mandate insurances to cover in vitro fertilization (IVF). The search may start by discovering which clinics accept their insurance.

Another consideration is location of the clinic. Because treatments often involve frequent short appointments for cycle monitoring, patients may want to consider one close to home or work. In some larger cities, offices may even offer early morning or lunchtime appointments to accommodate busy professionals. Patients inquiring about a clinic's success rate can research online at www.sartcorsonline.com. Encourage patients to be wary of reading online reviews, because they are likely to represent extremes. Many clinics host an open house that enables prospective patients to tour the facility and meet the doctors and staff, which can also include inquiring about financing options.

The initial visit with an REI is a lengthy consultation that involves reviewing the evaluation from the referring providers and likely includes a physical examination and ultrasound. The REI determines if any additional diagnostic tests are needed before making recommendations for treatments. For patients with anovulatory disorders, such as PCOS or hypothalamic amenorrhea, treatments may start with oral ovulation induction agents, such as clomiphene or letrozole (off-label) or injectable exogenous FSH, and engage in timed intercourse based on anticipated ovulation determined by follicle monitoring with serial ultrasounds. Intrauterine insemination (IUI) is a procedure similar to an endometrial biopsy, where a high concentration of sperm is injected into the uterus, usually in conjunction with triggered ovulation. It is another less-invasive alternative that may be offered for a few cycles before moving on to IVF.

There are some situations where IVF should be recommended as first-line therapy, such as for patients with bilateral tubal occlusions, severe male factor, or a serious uterine abnormality, although in that case a gestational carrier should be used. Because it is appreciated that the window for possible conception is narrow for women with DOR, an IVF cycle with a woman's own eggs should be attempted, although many women with DOR eventually seek IVF with donor eggs after failing to conceive with their own gametes. It becomes a trickier question with older women because younger age is the 1 factor that most predicts IVF success. Some clinicians believe it is reasonable to offer IVF as a first-line therapy to women over age 40, but most clinics impose an upper age limit on when they attempt an IVF cycle with the woman's own eggs. That average is 43 years, with a range of 41 year to 45 years. One study examined 231 women ages 45 to 49 who were doing IVF with their own eggs. Approximately one-third had the cycle canceled due to poor response, although there was a 21% pregnancy result. Only 5 of the 34 pregnancies achieved (2.1%) resulted in a live birth (all to women who were 45).[9] Thus, some clinics suggest IUIs to women over their own egg cutoff age because the success rates are similar to IVF, but IUI is less costly and less invasive.

The decision to accept donor gametes is a difficult one and a process that evolves over time. Many women experience a sense of disappointment; feelings of inadequacy and that their bodies have failed them, their partner, and their extended families. Patients need to grieve and come to terms with the loss that they will not pass on their own genetics to their children. Although many women who use donor eggs are able to make peace with the process as they get to experience a physiologic bond through pregnancy, men who need to use donor sperm sometimes feel isolated. This needs to be reconciled by the couple, and some couples seek adoption of a live born child or embryo adoption so that there is not a genetic disparity between the parents. Other heavy decisions that follow involve using a known donor (a sibling or other relative) or anonymous donor and discussing how to reveal the origin of conception to any future offspring.

So, what can patients expect when they are expecting an IVF cycle? The process usually starts by taking combination oral contraceptive pills or small doses of leuprolide to suppress any endogenous stimulation to the ovary. The REI creates a specific stimulation protocol based on a patient's age, antral follicle count, and AMH and FSH and E2 values, as well as any previous response to stimulation if applicable. The stimulant medications are administered as daily injections of exogenous FSH. For many women, this involves learning to administer their own injections. The duration of the stimulation cycle reflects the number of days in a natural cycle but varies depending on the stimulation protocol used and how a patient responds. During this time, patients go through follicle monitoring with serial transvaginal ultrasounds every other day and possibly every day toward the end of stimulation, when the REI is determining when to trigger ovulation and coordinate oocyte retrieval. The timing of the trigger is determined by follicular development, when numerous follicles are approximately 18 mm in size. Waiting too long can result in premature ovulation and some patients need to administer an antagonist (another injection) to prevent this occurrence. The trigger is meant to mimic the LH surge and to coordinate the retrieval 34 hours to 36 hours after the injection of recombinant human chorionic gonadotropin (hCG) or leuprolide. Women need to have flexibility with their schedules because procedure appointments can change suddenly based on the response to stimulation.

The egg or oocyte retrieval often takes place in conjunction with the laboratory where the eggs are fertilized and embryos cultured. Especially when there are a high number of follicles anticipated, general anesthesia may be used, but when fewer follicles are expected, lighter anesthetic options can be considered.

One of the main advantages of IVF is that it makes the process of human reproduction more efficient. Where a woman produces 1 or maybe 2 gametes each month during a natural cycle, the controlled hyperstimulation of her ovaries has allowed 10 or more oocytes to be aspirated into a needle that is inserted through the vagina under ultrasound guidance. Of all the oocytes that are retrieved, however, not all are mature and not all fertilized with sperm (either naturally or through intracytoplasmic sperm injection). Patients know how many mature oocytes were aspirated on the day of the retrieval and learn how many were successfully fertilized by the next day. The next decisions involve determining the timing and number of embryo transfers.

The 2 times to transfer an embryo are on the third day of embryologic development or on the fifth day. On the third day the embryos should be between 6 cells and 8 cells and the division should be uniform without minimal fragmentation. At the fifth day, the embryo is at the blastocyst stage. Not all day 3 embryos progress to the blastocyst stage, supporting a day 5 blastocyst transfer over a day 3 embryo transfer. Additionally, there is a grading system than can be applied to blastocysts to allow the embryologist to select the specimens that are most likely to result in a pregnancy. Similar pregnancy rates are achieved with transfers of fewer (1 or 2) blasts compared with transfers of multiple day 3 embryos, which still has the potential to result in multiple births.

Multiple gestations have become the burden of IVF success. Although the prospect of twins or even triplets is often welcomed by infertile couples, who may see multiple gestation as a more efficient way to create their family, it carries a high risk of mortality and morbidity due to previability and preterm deliveries. The other advantage of a day 5 transfer is that it allows for the opportunity for preimplantation genetic testing. Preimplantation genetic screening (PGS), sometimes referred to as comprehensive chromosomal screening, is a process of running a karyotype after performing a biopsy of the trophectoderm of the blastocyst. Preimplantation genetic diagnosis (PGD) involves the same biopsy process for obtaining cells from the blastocyst, but it tests for a specific gene mutation. For example, in a couple where both partners are carriers of cystic fibrosis, PGD can allow for selection of an unaffected embryo and avoid passing the condition onto their offspring. PGS and PGD are often used as interchangeable terms, but they have distinctive applications.

The premise of PGS is that by identifying which embryos are euploid (especially in a stimulation cycle that produced a high volume of embryos), the embryologist and REI can avoid transferring an abnormal embryo that would likely fail to implant, one that could result in an early miscarriage, or one whose abnormality would be discovered at the traditional time of genetic screening, forcing a couple to make some difficult decisions. It also revealed some of the limitations of the current systems for grading embryos, because many embryologist are surprised to learn that some embryos who earned high marks based on their appearance were chromosomally abnormal, and other receiving lower marks were euploid.

Although PGS seems to improve the pregnancy-per-embryo transfer rate, it has not demonstrated improvement in the overall birth rate from IVF procedures, because 1 study found that delivery rates were similar with a euploid single embryo transfer (eSET) versus a second transfer of an untested embryo if the first transfer of an untested embryo did not result in a live birth pregnancy.[10] Even though this approach does not change the overall birth rate, the benefits to a couple who may avoid the disappointment of a failed transfer and must endure the costs of an additional transfer or possible heartbreak of an early miscarriage are intangible.

The greatest potential for benefit with PGS may be reducing the rates of multiple gestations resulting from IVF. The Blastocyst Euploid Selective Transfer trial was the first randomized study to show that single embryo transfers could offer similar birth rates, while reducing the risks associated with a twin pregnancy. The study examined women who underwent an eSET and compared them with women doing an untested double embryo transfer (DET). The delivery rates were close (eSET 61% vs DET 65%), but the significant differences were in the rates of multiple gestation (eSET 0% vs 48%), which yielded a reduction in preterm birth (13% vs 29%) and reduced newborn ICU admissions associated with single-gestation pregnancies (11% vs 26%).[11]

The other consideration with a transfer of a day 5 embryo (even without doing PGS) is to select a fresh or frozen transfer. Over time, more evidence has shown improved pregnancy rates with transfer of a frozen embryo compared with fresh transfer. One theory is that a frozen transfer allows for more control and management of the uterine environment, which may be disorganized due to high E2 levels resulting from ovarian hyperstimulation. Although it is feared that some embryos will not survive the freezing and thawing process, it can be considered a good mark of quality for those that do. The other rationale for delaying the timing of the embryo transfer is to avoid ovarian hyperstimulation syndrome (OHSS). OHSS is a serious potential complication of ovarian stimulation and can lead to rapid fluid accumulation in the pelvis. In severe cases, patients can develop significant abdominal distention, weight gain, ascites, and pleural effusions. It can be fatal if not diagnosed in a timely manner and managed properly. The production of hCG from an early pregnancy can worsen OHSS, so avoiding a fresh transfer is often recommended for patients at risk of OHSS (women with PCOS or others who had a strong response to stimulation leading to a high number of oocytes retrieved and high estrogen levels).

After the transfer of a fresh or frozen embryo, patients can resume their usual activities. Although some clinics require patients to be on bed rest, it has not be shown to improve outcomes, and physical activity has not been demonstrated to be harmful. Especially in cases of a frozen transfer or donor egg cycle, exogenous progesterone needs to be administered in absence of endogenous production from a woman's ovaries. Again, different clinics vary in their protocols of how to administer progesterone (intramuscular, vaginal suppositories, tablets, gels, and rings) and for how long, but cessation typically occurs when it is perceived that the placenta has taken over the function of producing progesterone. Many REIs confirm pregnancy with a serum hCG level from 10 days to 14 days after the transfer. A negative result indicates a failed transfer and the patient should stop her luteal phase support. Patients with an ongoing pregnancy often have 1 or 2 ultrasounds with their REI to confirm viability (and number in cases of multiple embryo transfers) before graduating from their services and being referred to an obstetrician.

There are a few things to remember when caring for a now-pregnant infertile patient (or new mother by adoption). Infertility may have become a part of her identity and persist beyond pregnancy and parenting. She may have feeling of survivor's guilt, particularly if she bonded with other infertile women through a support group. She still has uncertainty about future pregnancies and may feel greedy about desiring more children. Pregnancy and adoption cure only childlessness, not infertility.

The other reality is that not all patients who are referred to a reproductive specialist return to the office with a pregnancy. What happens after a failed IVF cycle? Some patients attempt a second cycle, hoping to use the first cycle as a point for improvement. They may opt to seek a second opinion and fresh start with a new clinic. Patients with compromised gametes (DOR or severe male factor) may consider donor eggs or donor sperm. Patients may also consider donated embryos, using a gestational carrier, living without children, or adoption.

Tread lightly when raising the issue of adoption. Like the process of using donor gametes, the couple has to go through a process of mourning their loss of a genetic connection with their children. Adoption also carries additional emotional and physical baggage. Prospective parents must submit themselves to medical and psychiatric evaluations, fingerprinting and background checks, and multiple home study visits with a social worker. It also requires couples to answer personal questions about their own childhood and marriage as well as to produce documents, such as the 911 records and racial composition of their neighborhood, proof the septic tank can support another person, and a certificate of rabies vaccinations for pets. Then there are the decisions of open versus closed adoptions, domestic versus international adoptions I, and infant versus older child adoptions. Willingness to accept siblings or a child of a different race and being prepared for possible health problems, especially if a birth mother abused drugs during her pregnancy. Not to mention the fear of a birth mother changing her mind and deciding to parent herself before an adoption is finalized. Adoption can bear a price tag similar to IVF treatments.

SUMMARY

Infertility can be a daunting challenge for many couples. From the early stages of wondering if something is wrong, to a decision to take a step and get checked out, and to diving into the world of fertility treatments and hopefully to pregnancy and parenting, a resourceful, knowledgeable clinician can guide them through their journey.

REFERENCES

1. Guttenmacher AF. Journal American Medical Association 1956;65–503.
2. Gnoth C, Godehardt D, Godehard E, et al. Time to pregnancy: results of the German prospective study and impact on the management of infertility. Hum Reprod 2003;18:1959.
3. Speroff L, Glass RH, Kase NG. Clinical gynecologic endocrinology and infertility. 5th edition. 1994. p. 833.
4. Broekmans FJ, Kwee J, Hendriks DL, et al. A systematic review of tests predicating ovarian reserve and IVF outcome. Hum Reprod Update 2006;12:685.
5. Visser JA, de Jong FH, Laven JS, et al. Anti-Mullerian hormone review: a new marker for ovarian function. Reproduction 2006;131:1.

6. Luttjeboer F, Harada T, Hughes E, et al. Tubal flushing for subfertility. Cochrane Database Syst Rev 2007;(3):CD003718.
7. Cooper TG, Noonan E, von Eckardstein S, et al. World Health Organization reference values for human semen characteristics. Hum Reprod Update 2010;16:231.
8. Anawalt BD. Approach to male infertility: evaluation and induction of spermatogenesis. J Clin Endocrinol Metab 2013;98:3532.
9. Klipstein S, Regan M, Ryley DA, et al. One last chance for pregnancy: a review of 2705 IVF cycles initiated in women age 40 and above. Fertil Steril 2005;84:435.
10. Zang Z, Liu J, Collins GS, et al. Selection of single blastocysts for fresh transfer via standard morphology assessment alone and array CGH for good prognosis IVF patients: results from a randomized pilot study. Mol Cytogenet 2012;5:24.
11. Forman EJ, Scott RT. Euploid single embry transfer: the new IVF paradigm? Contemp Ob Gyn 2014.

Centering Pregnancy
A Novel Approach to Prenatal Care

Check for updates

Heather P. Adams, MPAS, PA-C[a,b,*], Carla Picardo, MD, MPH[b,c]

KEYWORDS

- Centering Pregnancy • Group prenatal care • Prenatal care • Centering

KEY POINTS

- The Centering Pregnancy model focuses on patient assessment and knowledge/education, with an added focus on patient support that distinguishes it from the traditional prenatal model.
- The Centering Pregnancy model empowers women by placing them in control of information used to assess not only their health but also the health of their fetus.
- Numerous studies have shown evidence of improved pregnancy outcomes with the use of Centering Pregnancy, particularly for culturally and socioeconomically high-risk populations.
- Education about the Centering Pregnancy model and awareness of the associated benefits may serve to address most if not all of the challenges associated with program implementation.
- Educational resources and tolls for implementation are accessible through the Centering Healthcare Institute.

INTRODUCTION

The dynamic characteristics of patients and their needs have prompted experiments in health care delivery; prenatal care is 1 example. The Centering Pregnancy model focuses on patient assessment and knowledge/education, similar to the traditional prenatal care, but adds a unique focus of patient support that addresses the physical, social, and emotional stressors of pregnancy through a group approach.[1] This innovative model offers prenatal care designed to empower women and their families, encourage interactive deliveries, offer comprehensive health care, and promote healthy behaviors. The original model for Centering Pregnancy was developed by

Disclosure Statement: The authors have no commercial or financial disclosures to report.
a Physician Assistant Department, Gannon University, 109 University Square, Erie, PA 16541, USA;
b Women's Wellness and Gynecology, 3939 West Ridge Road, Suite A-200, Erie, PA 16506, USA;
c Department of Obstetrics, Gynecology, and Reproductive Services, Magee-Womens Hospital of UPMC, 300 Halket Street, Pittsburgh, PA 15213, USA
* Corresponding author. Physician Assistant Department, Gannon University, 109 University Square, Erie, PA 16541.
E-mail address: Adams051@gannon.edu

nurse-midwife Sharon Schindler Rising in the 1990s.[2-4] Rising identified the need for a prenatal care model that focused on education, support, and personalized, culturally appropriate care.[2,4,5] This model was offered as an evidence-based alternative to traditional prenatal care, placing the emphasis on facilitated education rather than on structured lecturing by a provider.[6,7] This model has proved successful with various populations. Although it takes some effort to develop a Centering Pregnancy program, the benefits to patients, providers, and pregnancy outcomes are worth the effort.

THE CENTERING PREGNANCY MODEL

The Centering Pregnancy model of group prenatal care begins with a traditional pregnancy intake and initial 1-on-1 prenatal appointment; it includes a routine physical examination and collection of recommended cultures and bloodwork.[2,4] If a patient is medically low risk and elects to be part of the Centering Pregnancy program, she and her support person join a group of 8 to 12 pregnant women (and their supports) who have similar estimated dates of confinement. According to the curriculum material offered by the Centering Healthcare Institute, in Boston, Massachusetts, each group first meets between 12 weeks and 16 weeks of gestation, followed by 10 group sessions over 6 months, concluding with a postpartum visit.[3,4,7-9] Signed confidentiality agreements are required by all group members at the first group session to ensure security of personal information and encourage openness and willingness to share only within the group. Group session last 90 minutes to 120 minutes, and food/snacks should be available for participants.[2,4]

Because the Centering Pregnancy program includes the same physical assessment and education as traditional prenatal care, it meets the standards set forth by the American Congress of Obstetricians and Gynecologists and American Academy of Pediatrics.[4,10] It is recognized by Medicare and private health insurances, making billing comparable to traditional prenatal care visits through the standard reimbursement system.[7,10-12] The first 20 minutes to 45 minutes of each group visit begin as women arrive and measure and record their own weights and blood pressures. Some programs may also include a urine dipstick measurement for glucose and protein.[2-4] This model is believed to further empower women by placing them in control of information used to assess not only their health but also the health of their fetus. It may make specific medical evaluations more tangible to patients and stimulate questions and discussions about techniques and findings.[10] While women arrive and record their vital signs, each patient is systematically seen individually in a quieter, private area of the space by the medical provider for her assessment, physical examination (fundal height measurement and fetal heart tone auscultation), and discussion of concerns and/or questions. Examples of individual concerns include abnormal laboratory values, weight gain or loss, and psychosocial struggles. Individual questions brought to the facilitator's attention privately may be determined to benefit the entire group and guide the group discussion later in the session.[10] This private portion of the visit allows the provider to determine if additional laboratory tests, imaging, or individual appointments are needed. These additional visits occur within a traditional model in the office, but the patients continue with group appointments, unless deemed too medically high risk.[10,11]

While each woman meets privately with her health care provider, the remainder of the group has the opportunity to interact, bond, and complete a self-assessment sheet. The self-assessments introduce topics that will be discussed that day and are designed to gauge participants' knowledge on the subject as well as encourage the group to generate relevant questions and facilitate discussion.[4,10,11,13] The remainder of the appointment takes place in the group setting with participants arranged in a circle to illustrate all participants have equally important roles in the group. The locus of control is given to all patients/participants to have an active voice in the sessions.[14] Strategic discussion topics are presented based on gestation, and patients/supports are invited to ask questions that might benefit all group members. This format allows a dramatic increase in learning opportunities, resources, and support as group members share their own experiences and concerns, and discussion is guided by the trained health professional or guest experts in a facilitative rather than lecture approach.[4] The content of the educational topics designed to deliver optimal care and improve birth outcomes.[15] The Centering Pregnancy handbook outlines each class and corresponding information, so participants may read ahead, reflect, and prepare questions prior to each session/appointment.[16] **Table 1** lists common discussion topics, suggested gestational age in pregnancy for specific discussions, and potential expert guest speakers.

The facilitative design of Centering Pregnancy promotes open discussions in the group, decision making by patients, and bonding, allowing patients to ask questions they may otherwise hesitate to ask during a 1-on-1 traditional prenatal care visit.[6] The long-term relationships the provider forms with each individual and the group as a whole promote discussion of sensitive topics, including domestic violence.[5] Supplemental educational material, including handouts, brochures, interactive worksheets, and videos, may be incorporated.[4–6,10] Session summaries reinforce topics and serve as resources for women who missed a visit; for example, during a session about nutrition goals the group activity book may include a food diary and body mass index (BMI) chart.[4] Women would be encouraged to document their weight over time. This may promote goal setting regarding all aspects of healthy gestational weight: diet, exercise, and appropriate weight gain based on BMI.[9] Role playing and other group activities introduce concepts to teach women how to advocate for and voice their preferences, such as for labor analgesia and breastfeeding intentions.

Table 1 Suggestions for delivering the education component of center pregnancy group prenatal care		
Common Educational Topics for Centering Pregnancy Sessions	**Suggested Gestational Age**	**Possible Expert Speaker to Supplement Discussion**
Prenatal nutrition, fetal development, and the dangers of substance abuse	16 wk	Nutritionist
Common discomforts and changes to the female body during pregnancy	20 wk	Physical therapist
Exercise and relaxation during pregnancy	24 wk	Pregnancy yoga instructor
Family dynamics and intimate relations.	28 wk	Family psychologist
Infant feeding and coping strategies	30 wk	Lactation consultant
Birth plans and preparation for labor and delivery	32 wk	Labor and delivery nurse
Postpartum contraception	36 wk	Guest women's health care provider
Postpartum adjustment, postpartum depression, and care of the mother after delivery	38 wk	Nurse educator
Care of an infant and parenting strategies	40 wk	Social worker

Data from Refs.[3–5,10,15,17]

The Centering Pregnancy experience culminates with a postpartum visit and transitions into individual routine gynecologic care. The outcome of the Centering Pregnancy group experience is that women who may have had little in common other than their similar estimated dates of confinement have spent intensive time sharing experiences, supporting each other, and possibly developing ongoing relationships. Centering Pregnancy programs may facilitate continued contact between group members furthering the supportive, healthy relationships that developed.[12] In some locations, the group may transition into a Centering Pregnancy program that meets every few weeks to months for the first year of life of the newborns and provide well child checks and continued parenting education.

Centering Pregnancy gives patients more time with providers—20 hours of contact over the course of the pregnancy compared with an estimated 2 total hours of contact in a traditional prenatal care model.[5,7,10,18] The teaching model for Centering Pregnancy group prenatal care uses health care providers as facilitators at each group appointment. The facilitator may be a physician, midwife, or advanced practice clinician/provider who is trained and certified in the Centering Pregnancy model but may not be the same provider involved in the patient deliveries. The facilitator follows the same cohort of women throughout their pregnancies, improving continuity of care and contact time with the same provider.[5] Nurses, social workers, or health educators may fill the role of assistant facilitator.[5,15] One defining characteristic of this teaching style is flexibility because participants may steer the topics of discussion that may not always coincide with the planned curriculum, making this model process driven rather than content driven.[10,12] Novicks[14] found women identified 3 components they desire in prenatal care: continuity, comprehensiveness, and control. The Centering Pregnancy model is designed for 1 consistent provider and assistant to facilitate all prenatal sessions. The topics are comprehensive and the amount of time spent on each topic is driven by the women in the group, thus meeting all 3 patient-desired components.[14,16]

BENEFITS OF CENTERING PREGNANCY

A group approach to health care has been used successfully in several areas of clinical medicine, such as diabetes, geriatrics, and pediatrics, and has been associated with many benefits. These include community building, a sense of support, exposure to problem-solving skills, improved self-esteem, and an increase in clinical knowledge and healthy behaviors. These benefits lead to higher patient satisfaction, improved quality of life, and a decrease in acute care visits, all while efficiently and cost-effectively using facilities and resources.[11,15] Benefits likely stem from the empowerment, education, and active participation central to group care.[12] Centering Pregnancy as a model of group care has resulted in many of these same benefits. Experiences with group prenatal care show health care provider continuity, personalized care, inclusion of family support structure, encouragement of lifelong healthy behaviors, and improved attendance rates all at a cost similar to traditional care. An increase in medical knowledge and decrease in anxiety among patients may occur.[1]

Some studies have shown improvements in pregnancy outcomes with participation in group prenatal care. These include lower rates of preterm delivery and low birthweight and an increase in breastfeeding rates, patient satisfaction with prenatal care, knowledge, family planning and sexually transmitted infection prevention behaviors, and preparedness for labor and delivery.[6,15,18–20] **Table 2** summarizes studies comparing pregnancy outcomes of patients who participated in Centering Pregnancy group prenatal care and traditional prenatal care. These studies span from the inception of Centering Pregnancy in 1998 through 2017 and include data from studies

Table 2
Summary of studies comparing various pregnancy outcomes of Centering Pregnancy and traditional prenatal care

Study	Study Design	Population/Sample Size	Outcomes Centering Pregnancy	Outcomes Traditional Prenatal Care	P Value
Rising,[4] 1998	Observational	111 Ethnically diverse, primarily Medicaid insured women	• Preterm delivery, 4.5% • Low birthweight, 5.4% • Third-trimester ED visits, 26%	• No results reported • No results reported • Third-trimester ED visits, 74%	— — .001
Grady & Bloom,[21] 2004	Retrospective chart review	Adolescents 124 Centering 144 Regular care (2001) 233 Regular care (1998)	• No show rate, 19% • Preterm delivery, 10.5% • Low birthweight, 8.9% • C/S rate, 13.7% • Self-reported breastfeeding rate, 46% • Patient identified pediatrician prior to discharge, 79%	• No show rate, 28% • Preterm delivery, 25.7%/23.2% (2001/1998) • Low birthweight, 22.9%/18.3% (2001/1998) • C/S rate, 14.6/15.9% (2001/1998) • Self-reported breastfeeding rate, 28% (1998 only) • Patient identified pediatrician prior to discharge, 52% (1998 only)	Not published <.02/<.05 (2001/1998) <.02/<.05 (2001/1998) >.05 <.02 <.02
Ickovics et al,[15] 2003	Prospective matched cohort Matched by clinic, age, race, parity, and infant birth date	Low income mostly African American and Hispanic women at public clinics in Atlanta, GA, and New Haven, CT 229 Centering 229 Regular care	• Average birthweight, 3228.2 g • Preterm <33 wk, 0.9% • Preterm 33–36.9 wk, 8.3% • Low birthweight (<2500 g), 7% • Very low birthweight (<1500 g), 1.3% • Neonatal deaths, 0%	• Average birthweight, 3159.1 g • Preterm <33 wk, 3.1% • Preterm 33–36.9 wk 6.5% • Low birthweight (<2500 g), 10% • Very low birthweight (<1500 g), 2.6% • Neonatal deaths, 1.3%	<.01 .83 .38 NA NA NA

(continued on next page)

Table 2
(continued)

Study	Study Design	Population/Sample Size	Outcomes Centering Pregnancy	Outcomes Traditional Prenatal Care	P Value
Ickovics et al,[20] 2007	RCT	Mostly African American women at public clinics in Atlanta, GA, and New Haven, CT 623 Centering 370 Regular care	• Preterm births, 9.8% • Preterm births among African Americans, 10% • Low birthweight (<2500 g), 11.3% • Breastfeeding initiation, 66.5% • Prenatal knowledge score, 41.1 • Readiness score for labor and delivery, 76.2 • Readiness score for infant care, 90.0 • Satisfaction with PNC score, 113.3 • Mean cost for PNC, $4149 • Mean cost for delivery, $3433	• Preterm births, 13.8% • Preterm births among African Americans, 15.8% • Low birthweight (<2500 g), 10.7% • Breastfeeding initiation, 54.6% • Prenatal knowledge score, 38.5 • Readiness score for labor and delivery, 68.6 • Readiness score for infant care, 86.9 • Satisfaction with PNC score, 108.4 • Mean cost for PNC, $4091 • Mean cost for delivery, $3417	.045 .02 .90 .001 <.001 <.001 .056 <.001 .69 .94
Kennedy et al,[22] 2011	RCT	224 Women from 2 military settings >50% White >50% Married	• Attended <9 visits, 12.9% • Preterm birth, 7.8% • Low birthweight (<2500 g), 4.6% • NICU admission, 8.9% • Epidural use, 74.2%	• Attended <9 visits, 46.7% • Preterm birth, 5.5% • Low birthweight (<2500 g), 4.6% • NICU admission, 3.7% • Epidural use, 57.9%	<.01 .46 1.00 .19 <.01

Study	Design	Population	Centering	Regular care	P value
Ickovics et al,[23] 2016	Cluster RCT	Mostly Latina and African American adolescent women from 14 health centers in New York City, NY — 573 Centering, 575 Regular care	• Preterm birth 10.1% • Low birthweight (<2500 g), 8.7% • Small for gestational age, 11% • Breastfeeding initiation, 88.8% • NICU admission, 15.4%	• Preterm birth 10.1% • Low birthweight (<2500 g), 9.8% • Small for gestational age, 15.8% • Breastfeeding initiation, 87.2% • NICU admission, 17.3%	NS NS .04 NS NS
Kominiarek et al,[9] 2017	Retrospective cohort study	Low-income, mostly urban women in Greenville, SC, matched 1:2 with women with similar BMI, insurance, and gestational age at delivery — 2117 Centering, 4234 Regular care	• 4% Gestational diabetes • Mean weight gain below recommendations, 20% • Mean weight gain exceeding recommendations, 55% • Preterm delivery, 7% • Mean birthweight, 3250 g ± 523	• 6% Gestational diabetes • Mean weight gain below recommendations, 26% • Mean weight gain exceeding recommendations, 48% • Preterm delivery, 5.8% • Mean birthweight, 3285 g ± 524	$P = .005$ — $P < .001$ .04 .01

Abbreviations: CS, cesarean section; ED, emergency department; NA, numbers too small to calculate P value/statistical testing; NS, P value not significant (ie, >.05); PNC, prenatal care.

involving vulnerable populations. Some studies show statistically significant improvement in various pregnancy outcomes, and all show no evidence of harm caused by this model of prenatal care.

A recent meta-analysis by Carter and colleagues[17] is a comprehensive review of the literature comparing group prenatal care (N = 3229) and traditional prenatal care (N = 7092). Ultimately 4 randomized controlled trials (RCTs) and 10 observational studies were included in their analysis of the effect of care model on preterm delivery, low birthweight, neonatal ICU (NICU) admissions, and breastfeeding. The studies were heterogeneous and in 8 of them prior rates of preterm births were not reported in either comparison group. Of the 10 observational studies, only 3 met the criteria for high quality. The rate of preterm birth was statistically significantly lower among African American women in group prenatal care when the pooled analysis was limited to the high-quality studies (8% vs 11.1%). This translates to a reduction of 3 preterm births per 100 live births in African American women. Nine of the studies, including all RCTs, reported lower rates of low birthweight in the group model (7.5% vs 9.5%); this effect disappeared when only RCTs were pooled and analyzed (7.9% vs 8.7%). There were no significant differences between the groups in NICU admissions or breastfeeding uptake. This systematic review concluded there was no evidence group prenatal care caused harm. It also underscored that Centering Pregnancy may have more benefits for some social, ethnic, and economic groups.[17]

It is widely recognized that women in certain circumstances may experience additional and unique challenges with pregnancy and prenatal care. These populations include adolescents, women from various cultures, and women in unstable relationships. Maternal and infant mortality rates are higher in African American women compared with non-Hispanic white women. African American women show a rate of preterm birth double that of white women, even after correcting for socioeconomic discrepancies, highlighting the potential impact group prenatal care may have on this population of women.[17] Hispanic women often share similar socioeconomic circumstances as African American women.[11] The Latina paradox, however, may be responsible for their lower rates of preterm births and less robust benefits from group care. Despite similar economic stressors, it is proposed the benefits of the Latina community structure and family support trump other influences.[17,24] Certain poor pregnancy outcomes, such as low birthweight and preterm delivery, are often higher among the vulnerable population of adolescents.[12,21] Centering Pregnancy offers not only a welcoming environment for these young women with their peers but also a schedule such that transportation issues and class absences may be minimized with evening or weekend groups. The supportive and educational components of Centering Pregnancy may make this model ideal for these populations, offering a superior method of delivering prenatal care to populations of women who are marginalized by socioeconomic status, race, or culture.[1,11]

CHALLENGES AND LIMITATIONS OF CENTERING PREGNANCY

A key factor that influences the success of Centering Pregnancy programs is openness of patients, health professionals, and clinic staff to a new model of prenatal care. This includes the ability to address scheduling challenges, allocation of resources, and staff/provider buy-in, particularly for employees who are not directly involved in the implementation of the program but may be affected by its existence in the workplace.[18] For success, this model of care must not be seen as inferior to the traditional model. Additionally, both providers and patients must be comfortable with the facilitator role of the health care provider.[10]

Several barriers or limitations of the Centering Pregnancy model have been discussed. Some critics do not believe women are receiving the same depth and breadth of medical care as with a traditional prenatal model.[2] There are concerns about maintenance of patient confidentiality/Health Insurance Portability and Accountability Act of 1996 compliance as well as lack of individualized attention. For some practices that are interested in starting a Centering Pregnancy program, creating a 2-hour block of availability for a healthcare provider to facilitate group may be difficult. In this situation, providers in the obstetric group practice may assume a negative opinion of the program because a colleague has been removed from the practice schedule to facilitate a group while they remain in clinic with a full schedule of patients with various concerns and complaints. There may be a lack of knowledge about billing the group visits during the program's infancy.[1,2] Additional challenges of this model include patient and provider discomfort with the facilitator role and group format, feelings about the meeting space and snacks provided, and patients possibly not meeting the provider who will deliver their babies.[1,10] The group model does not typically support the attendance of children of the mothers involved. Childcare during the longer visits could be a challenge for some women.[16] Other patient populations may experience unique challenges. For example, due to transient populations and frequent relocation of patients and trained providers, military populations have identified difficulty in achieving the following with the Centering Pregnancy model: adequate staffing, allocation and maintenance of financial resources and space, availability of childcare during visits, time needed for recruitment efforts, and adequate leadership commitment to the program.[16]

Vonderbeid and colleagues[7] performed a qualitative descriptive study using focus groups involving 35 participants to identify challenges of Centering Pregnancy implementation and patient retention. The specific challenges were categorized into those identified by patients, providers and ancillary staff, and administrators. Investigators coupled this with social marketing strategies and suggestions to address each challenge. These challenges and potential solutions are summarized in **Table 3**. Although this study identified potential obstacles to Centering Pregnancy programming, the list of suggested solutions indicates education about the model and awareness of benefits may address these challenges. Additionally, data consistently show there are many benefits with this model and no evidence that Centering Pregnancy causes harm, indicating any efforts necessary to overcome challenges are worthwhile.[15,17,19,20]

IMPLEMENTATION OF CENTERING PREGNANCY PROGRAMS

Recent health care reform has prompted providers and health care facilities to discover new and innovative ways to offer cost-efficient, effective, quality care. Centering Pregnancy care fits these standards.[4,7] This model is adaptable to a variety of health care settings evidenced by successful implementation in the United States, Canada, Australia, the United Kingdom, and countries in Africa.[18] Starting a Centering Pregnancy program involves knowledge of resources and the training and certification processes. The Centering Healthcare Institute is a 501(c)(3) nonprofit organization that provides resources for patients and health care providers about the program, including implementation. Certain requirements are necessary for program accreditation by the Centering Healthcare Institute.[2,4,6,7,16] Resources are accessible at www.centeringhealthcare.org.

The Centering Pregnancy model of prenatal care has proved an effective and efficient use of providers' time without expensive modifications or equipment. It does require provisions for adequate space.[4,7,10,16,18] The designated space must allow

Table 3
Challenges to implementation of Centering Pregnancy and proposed solutions identified by Vonderbeid and colleagues[7]

Challenges for Patients	Proposed Solutions
Lack of privacy and confidentiality	Inform women they will have individual time with the provider at the beginning of every appointment.
Change in the patient-provider relationship	Assure each patient her relationship with the provider remains a focus of this model.
Lack of understanding of the group care model	Describe the group sessions and the specific benefits of this model.
Logistics including time, preparation conflicts, childcare, language barriers, and appointment length	Reassure appointments begin and end on time and explain the total prenatal time in the office may not change but time with the provider will increase.

Challenges for Providers and Ancillary Staff	Proposed Solutions
Lack of understanding of this model and its benefits	Provide literature on this model and invite providers to observe a group in action.
Concerns of decreased productivity	Provide data about the potential for increased productivity by seeing 8–12 patients in a 2-h timeframe and reassure providers these visits are reimbursed.
Changes to the patient-provider relationship	Provide data on improvements in health outcomes and in patient satisfaction.
Need for preparation and teamwork	Offer gratitude to staff for the efforts, necessary for a successful program and reinforce increased patient satisfaction.

Challenges for Administrators	Proposed Solutions
Revenue, cost, and productivity, including cost of ongoing training	Share the role of the program to market the entire practice. Reassure the visits are reimbursed (sometimes at a higher rate) and highlight improvements in patient satisfaction and outcomes.
Space availability	Encourage the potential to turn a non–revenue-generating group space into a revenue generating space.

From Vonderbeid SC, Klima CS, Norr KF, et al. Using focus groups and social marketing to strengthen promotion of group prenatal care. ANS Adv Nurs Sci 2013;36(4):325–31; with permission.

facilitative participation by all group members. Enough room is needed to provide an open but private area in the space where individual assessments take place, an area for a large circle of chairs for "Circling Up" during the remainder of the session, and accessible bathrooms.[16] Furthermore, program success requires support and recruitment efforts by more than just those directly involved in the program. Administrative, provider, and staff support for the program is integral to its success.[2]

SUMMARY

The Centering Pregnancy model offers a unique experience for both participants and health care providers. The group design promotes community building and development of a support structure as well as improvement in patient insight, apathy, and problem-solving skills.[4] Women are welcome to participate in Centering Pregnancy, regardless of their birth plan, relationship status, plans for breastfeeding, or other views about pregnancy and the postpartum period. The main focus is to remove the authoritative style of prenatal care and empower women to control their own, fetal, and newborn health and well-being.[2] Evidence of the benefits of Centering Pregnancy are compelling; there are several robust studies, including RCTs, identifying similar or improved obstetric, reproductive, and public health outcomes, particularly for culturally and socioeconomically high-risk populations, and high rates of both patient and provider satisfaction[4,9,15,16,20–23] Challenges for Centering Pregnancy programs exist, but suggested solutions to such challenges are straightforward, involving staff education and increased communication of benefits to patients, providers, and practices that chose to offer this model of care.[7] There is no evidence in the literature that Centering Pregnancy is associated with patient harm or worse health outcomes.[17] All these factors support the use of Centering Pregnancy as a novel approach to prenatal care and indicate that it can have a positive impact the experience of pregnancy, delivery, and motherhood in a meaningful way.

REFERENCES

1. Herrman JW, Rogers S, Ehrenthal DB. Women's perceptions of Centering Pregnancy: a focus group study. MCN Am J Matern Child Nurs 2012; 37(1):19–26.
2. Bell KM. Centering Pregnancy: changing the system, empowering women and strengthening families. Int J Childbirth Educ 2012;27(1):70–6.
3. McCartney PR. Centering Pregnancy: a renaissance in prenatal care? MCN Am J Matern Child Nurs 2004;29:261.
4. Rising SS. Centering Pregnancy: an interdisciplinary model of empowerment. J Nurse Midwifery 1998;43(1):46–54.
5. Carlson NS, Lowe NK. Centering Pregnancy: a new approach to prenatal care. MCN Am J Matern Child Nurs 2006;31(4):218–23.
6. Hartman S, D'Cunha M, Kolasa-Lenarz A, et al. Meeting the ACGME milestones through group prenatal care. Family Doctor 2015;3(4):23–6.
7. Vonderbeid SC, Klima CS, Norr KF, et al. Using focus groups and social marketing to strengthen promotion of group prenatal care. ANS Adv Nurs Sci 2013; 36(4):320–35.
8. Hale N, Picklesimer AH, Billings DL, et al. The impact of Centering Pregnancy group prenatal care on postpartum family planning. Am J Obstet Gynecol 2014;50:e1–7.
9. Kominiarek MA, Crockett A, Covington-Kolb S, et al. Association of group prenatal care with gestational weight gain. Obstet Gynecol 2017;129(4):663–70.
10. Reid J. Centering Pregnancy: a model for group prenatal care. Nurs Womens Health 2007;11(4):383–8.
11. Robertson B, Aycock DM, Darnell LA. Comparison of Centering Pregnancy to traditional care in Hispanic mothers. Matern Child Health J 2009;13:407–14.
12. Klima CS. Centering Pregnancy: a model for pregnant adolescents. J Midwifery Womens Health 2003;48(3):220–5.
13. Shakespeare K, Waite PJ, Gast J. A comparison of health behaviors of women in Centering Pregnancy and traditional prenatal care. Matern Child Health J 2010; 14:202–8.
14. Novicks G. Women's experience of prenatal care: an integrative review. J Midwifery Womens Health 2009;54(3):226–37.

15. Ickovics JR, Kershaw TS, Westdahl C, et al. Group prenatal care and preterm birth weight: results from a matched cohort study at public clinics. Obstet Gynecol 2003;102(5):1051–7.
16. Foster GA, Alviar A, Neumeier R, et al. A tri-service perspective on the implementation of a Centering Pregnancy model in the military. J Obstet Gynecol Neonatal Nurs 2012;41:315–21.
17. Carter EB, Temming LA, Akin J, et al. Group prenatal care compared with traditional prenatal care: a systematic review and meta-analysis. Obstet Gynecol 2016;128(3):551–61.
18. Kania-Richmond A, Hetherington E, McNeil D, et al. The impact of introducing Centering Pregnancy in a community health setting: a qualitative study of experiences of health center clinical and support staff. Matern Child Health J 2017;21: 1327–35.
19. Byerley BM, Haas DM. A systematic overview of the literature regarding group prenatal care for high-risk pregnancy women. BMC Pregnancy Childbirth 2017; 17:329.
20. Ickovics JR, Kershaw TS, Westdahl C, et al. Group prenatal care and perinatal outcomes: a randomized controlled trial. Obstet Gynecol 2007;110(2):330–9.
21. Grady MA, Bloom KC. Pregnancy outcomes of adolescents enrolled in a Centering Pregnancy program. J Midwifery Womens Health 2004;49(5):412–20.
22. Kennedy HP, Farrell T, Paden R, et al. A randomized clinical trial of group prenatal care in two military settings. Mil Med 2011;176(10):1169–77.
23. Ickovics JR, Earnshaw V, Lewis JB, et al. Cluster randomized controlled trial of group prenatal care: Perinatal outcomes among adolescents in New York City health centers. Am J Public Health 2016;106(2):359–65.
24. McGlade MS, Somnath S, Dahlstrom ME. The latina paradox: an opportunity for restructuring prenatal care delivery. Am J Public Health 2004;94(12):2062–5.

The Role of Pelvic Floor Physical Therapy for the Female Patient

Kristen M. Murphy, PT, DPT[a],*,
Aleece Fosnight, MSPAS, PA-C, CSC, CSE[b]

KEYWORDS

- Pelvic floor • Pelvic pain • Physical therapy • Incontinence • Dyspareunia
- Pelvic evaluation

KEY POINTS

- As the understanding of female pelvic floor dysfunction expands, both in a general sense and as it relates to pregnancy, there is an ever-growing need to recognize the important role that physical therapists can play in the support of regular obstetric and gynecologic care.
- Physical therapy has many benefits and is a less-invasive and well-tolerated supplement to traditional medical interventions for obstetric and gynecologic patients.
- Understanding the role that these practitioners can play in the recovery and treatment process can be a valuable addition to the patient's team of allies. Prevention and early intervention through a physical therapist can be effective in reducing the patient's risk for many of the diagnoses discussed.

INTRODUCTION

As the understanding of female pelvic floor dysfunction expands, both in a general sense and as it relates to pregnancy, there is an ever-growing need to recognize the important role that physical therapists (PTs) can play in the support of regular obstetric and gynecologic care. The purpose of this article is to impart a deeper understanding and awareness of the bony and pelvic floor muscle (PFM) anatomy, the physical therapy examination of the PFM, and commonly seen diagnoses that can be helped by physical therapy.

ANATOMY

The bones of the pelvis consist of the sacrum, coccyx, and 2 innominate bones.[1] The innominate is formed by the joining of the ilium, ischium, and pubis with the central

Disclosure: The authors of this article have no conflict of interest or financial disclosure.
[a] Perfect Balance Physical Therapy, 59 Oakdale Street, Brevard, NC 28712, USA; [b] Pisgah Urology, 87 Medical Park Drive, Suite A, Brevard, NC 28712, USA
* Corresponding author.
E-mail address: kristenmurphydpt@gmail.com

Physician Assist Clin 3 (2018) 445–455
https://doi.org/10.1016/j.cpha.2018.02.011
2405-7991/18/© 2018 Elsevier Inc. All rights reserved.

physicianassistant.theclinics.com

fusion point being the acetabulum. The bony anatomy of the pelvis creates the framework for the support and function of the muscular pelvic floor and abdomen. Within the pelvis, there is an inherent stability secondary to the structural formation of the sacroiliac joint and the pubic symphysis. The structure here helps to establish the form closure of these joints creating a solid platform on which to build.

The ligamentous support of the lumbopelvic-hip complex is vast and serves to create even further stability. Although there are many significant ligaments in this region, the sacrotuberous[2] and sacrospinous[3] ligaments are the 2 most commonly associated with pain, limitations, and neural dysfunction (**Fig. 1**).

The PFMs are divided into 3 layers and are discussed from the most superficial to the deepest. Within layer 1 will be found the bulbocavernosus (also called bulbospongiosus), ischiocavernosus, superficial transverse perineal, and external anal sphincter muscles[1] (**Fig. 2**).

Layer 2 is commonly associated with layer 1 because it underlies the first layer in a very similar arrangement. Here, the deep transverse perineal, sphincter urethrovaginalis, compressor urethra, and external urethral sphincter muscles are located within the perineal membrane[1] (**Fig. 3**). The first 2 layers are commonly considered to be the "closer" muscles, and the primary function is sphincteric control for continence and sexual appreciation.[3]

Within layer 3 are found the levator ani group (pubococcygeus and iliococcygeus muscles) and the coccygeus muscles (**Fig. 4**). This layer is considered the "lifter" muscles, and the primary function of layer 3 is support of the internal pelvic organs, vagina,[4] and rectum.

Although not directly part of the PFM, the obturator internus (OI) and piriformis muscles are associated with PFM function and dysfunction. The OI forms the anterolateral wall of the pelvis, and the iliococcygeus of the levator ani attaches to it laterally via the

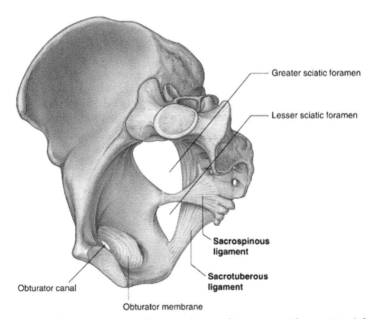

Greater sciatic foramen

Lesser sciatic foramen

Sacrospinous ligament

Sacrotuberous ligament

Obturator canal

Obturator membrane

Fig. 1. Location of sacrospinous and sacrotuberous ligaments with associated foraminal openings. (*From* Drake RL, Vogl AW, Mitchell A. Pelvis and perineum. In: Gray's anatomy for students. 3rd edition. Elsevier: Philadelphia; 2015. p. 450; with permission.)

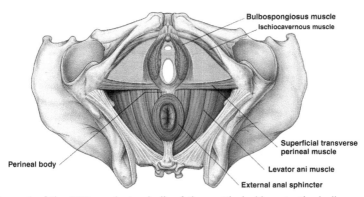

Fig. 2. Layer 1 of the PFM overlaying bulb of the vestibule (deep to the bulbospongiosus) and crus of the clitoris (deep to ischiocavernosus). (*From* Drake RL, Vogl AW, Mitchell A. Pelvis and perineum. In: Gray's anatomy for students. 3rd edition. Elsevier: Philadelphia; 2015. p. 439; with permission.)

arcus tendinous levator ani. The piriformis forms part of the posterior wall and sand-wiches the sciatic nerve between it and the OI.

The innervation of the pelvis and perineum arises from as high as T12 down to S5. The thoracolumbar contributions contribute to the motor and sensory function of the external genitalia and the hip/thigh/lower abdomen.[5] The sacral levels provide the innervation to the PFM via the levator ani nerve (S3-5) and the pudendal nerve (S2-4) primarily.

PHYSICAL THERAPY EVALUATION OF THE PELVIC FLOOR

A thorough PT evaluation of pelvic dysfunction should include history review, assess-ing lumbopelvic rhythm functionally (range of motion and stability in standing), bony alignment of the lumbopelvic-hip complex, abdominal and pelvic palpation, external

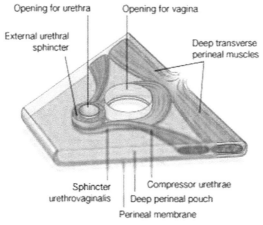

Fig. 3. Layer 2 of the PFM within the perineal membrane. (From Drake RL, Vogl AW, Mitchell A. Pelvis and perineum. In: Gray's anatomy for students. 3rd edition. Elsevier: Philadelphia; 2015. p. 459; with permission.)

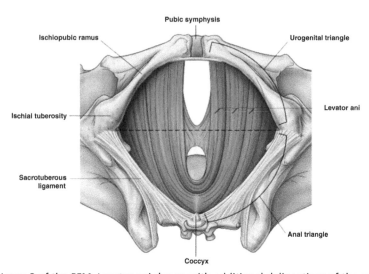

Fig. 4. Layer 3 of the PFM. Levator ani shown with additional delineations of the pubococcygeus (pubovaginalis and puborectalis) with iliococcygeus most laterally. Coccygeus obscured by the sacrotuberous ligament. (*From* Drake RL, Vogl AW, Mitchell A. Pelvis and perineum. In: Gray's anatomy for students. 3rd edition. Elsevier: Philadelphia; 2015. p. 503; with permission.)

observation of the perineum, neurologic screening, and strength testing of the hips, abdomen, and PFM, and internal PFM assessment (discussed later).

Unlike a traditional medical pelvic examination, only one digit will be used to assess the form and function of the PFM, ligaments, fascia, and nerves of the pelvis intravaginally or intrarectally depending on the patient's primary complaint. The following is a step-wise progression through the PT pelvic examination and assessment.

External examination is conducted to assess for any anomalies in coloration, tissue integrity/turgor, visible scars/deformities, perineal positioning, visible evidence of prolapse, and notable infection/lesions that would contraindicate an internal examination.

Internal examination of the PFM is used to determine muscle tone at rest, muscle integrity, voluntary and involuntary contractions, and excursion of the PFM. The internal assessment begins with insertion of the digit to the first knuckle using the introitus as the landmark for depth. At this level of insertion, one would assess the layer 1 muscles for tone looking for symmetry from right to left and anterior to posterior. The patient would be directed to complete a voluntary contraction, and the PT will assess for strength and quality of the contraction, typically felt as a "squeeze" to the digit.

Insertion to the level of the second knuckle will now allow for assessment of the layer 2 muscles. Assessment will be like that of layer 1, but the patient may be cued to "pretend you are stopping the flow of urine." The PT will again be feeling for a "squeeze" around the digit, felt mostly at 1 and 11 o'clock.

Layer 3 will be assessed with the digit fully inserted. Right and left halves should be assessed for symmetry of tone, fiber alignment, scar tissue, and so forth. Ligaments and fascia will also be most fully assessed at this depth, and OI can be palpated lateral to the levator ani on the side wall. The PT can assess the strength of the PFM in their entirety with full insertion. The Laycock scale[6] is most commonly used when grading the PFM strength (**Table 1**).

Table 1	
Label: description of the grading for pelvic floor muscle strength in a pelvic floor evaluation	
Laycock's "Modified Oxford Scale"	
Grade	**Description**
0: Zero	No palpable contraction
1: Trace	Flicker or pulsation
2: Poor	Contraction with no lift
3: Fair	Moderate contraction with lift posterior > anterior
4: Good	Contraction and lift with compression from anterior, posterior, and side walls
5: Strong	Stronger lift and compression with cephalic lift of the digit with resistance against posterior vaginal wall

Adapted from Laycock J, Jerwood D. Pelvic floor muscle assessment: the PERFECT scheme. Physiotherapy 2001;87(12);633; with permission.

COMMON DIAGNOSES ADDRESSED WITH PHYSICAL THERAPY
Low Back and Sacroiliac Joint Pain

It has been shown that low back pain and instability are common among pregnant women with some studies finding prevalence as high as 72% of women suffering with it to some degree.[7] It is thought that the release of relaxin during later stages of pregnancy can contribute to this high prevalence.[8] Relaxin is also released during the luteal phase of the menstrual cycle and is associated with higher prevalence of pain during this time.[9] Although the opening of the pelvic outlet and the softening of the joints of the pelvic ring are important and necessary for delivery, the instability created can lead to many issues for patients. Proper pelvic alignment is important not only for decreasing the pain associated with this opening but also with proper functioning of the PFM. Appropriate stability training can be effective in improving pain complaints and inherent control. Targeted stability training for activation of the inner core (PFM and transverse abdominus) with coactivation of hip and spinal muscles was found effective in reducing pain and improving function.[10] The addition of manual therapy for joint mobilization, soft tissue releases, or stretching can also provide additional benefit. When necessary, external support, such as a sacroiliac belt or pregnancy support belt, may be used temporarily until the inner core strength improves enough to overcome the instability.

Diastasis Recti Abdominis

The separation of the rectus abdominis (RA) muscles is a significant concern during and following pregnancy. With a prevalence as high as 52% among patients seeking urogynecologic care, this issue is large one. Many of these patients may not have notable symptoms of the diastasis recti abdominis (DRA) but will present with a comorbid pelvic floor diagnosis, such as urinary incontinence (UI), fecal incontinence (FI), or pelvic organ prolapse (POP).[11]

Targeted exercises focusing on the inner core and RA activation can be beneficial in reducing the risk of DRA and improving the separation after pregnancy. Pregnant women who exercised were found by one study to have a prevalence of 12.5% as opposed to nonexercisers with a prevalence of 90%.[12] If the separation is more chronic in nature, it may be necessary to release the fascia of the lateral abdomen allowing for strengthening and weight-transfer training to become more effective. Letting the fascia stay shortened will decrease the likelihood of success with reducing the DRA with exercise alone.

Round Ligament Pain

The round ligaments of the uterus originate at the horns of the uterus, travel through the inguinal canal, and then insert at the labia majora overlying the pubic bone. During the second and third trimester, the round ligament of the uterus will stretch considerably from the size of a pinky to the length of a pencil and thin in width considerably. This stretching can cause significant pain in the lower abdomen and groin, most notably with quick movements such as coughing, reaching, rising from a chair, or rolling over in bed. The pain is most often unilateral with a short, sharp catch, which will ease after a few moments; however, if the ligament becomes spastic, the pain can last for longer periods.

Education on body mechanics for proper movement patterns, avoiding twisting, care with lifting, and generally being slow about movements will be addressed by a PT. Strengthening of the abdominal muscles can help to limit the stress on the ligaments and decrease the pain from the ongoing tension.[13] Manual therapy to the spastic ligament and application of heat can reduce the pain and assist in the progressive lengthening of the ligament.

Birth Trauma Causing Pelvic Organ Prolapse, Urinary Incontinence, and Fecal Incontinence

Trauma to the PFM, fascia, or other support structures during childbirth is associated with a decrease in the uterine support and overall function of the PFM. These deficits will often lead to varying amounts of UI, FI, or POP. There is growing evidence showing that disruption of the rectovaginal septum during delivery results in higher prevalence of true rectocele and obstructive defecation.[14] Levator ani trauma is linked with increased likelihood of UI and POP. Women with these conditions have been found to have a decrease in levator muscle volume as well as increased levator hiatus width.[14] Levator avulsion has been found in 25% of women with uterine descent and in about 50% of women with second- or third-degree uterine prolapse. There is also a link between levator ani trauma and stress UI in the first 3 months postpartum, but this is less true later in life, although there is a higher likelihood of trauma for women who have their first child at a later age. Age is important to keep in mind given that in the United States the age of primiparae continues to increase.

In the case of PFM trauma and subsequent symptoms, there is a great deal that PT can do to help decrease symptoms. Following an assessment to determine the extent of the damage or weakness, a program can be initiated to improve the function of the PFM. Supervised PFM retraining to elicit proper contraction and coordination of the PFM should be initiated once cleared by the physician to return to normal activity.

Physical therapy will help with symptoms of urogenital prolapse but in most cases will have minimal effect on the topographic changes present. POP is also best treated with strengthening as a first intervention[15] or as a preoperative option for patients who necessitate surgical intervention. There is a significant benefit to patients who undergo preoperative physical therapy as compared with those who do not with respect to urinary symptoms, quality of life, and PFM strength postoperatively.[16]

A strengthening program will include exercises for the lumbopelvic-hip complex with focus on PFM activation[15] with functional mobility.[17] It has been found that a combination of general PFM strength training and precontraction (or knack) training before increases in abdominal pressure should both be integral in a PFM training program. It was found in one study that targeted strengthening was effective in improving uncontrolled urine loss by as much as 38% in 1 week and 74% after 1 month.[18] If needed, PFM electrical stimulation or biofeedback training may be used to improve muscle function when voluntary contraction is not sufficient or to improve patient understanding/control.

Urge UI can also be effectively treated with a strengthening program, but there needs to be a significant component of behavioral training as well. Patients need to be educated on dietary contributions to urgency and UI, namely avoidance of caffeine and other bladder irritants.[15] Bladder retraining using urgency suppression through PFM contraction and the spinal reflex arc can decrease the sense of urgency to assist in lengthening voiding intervals. The success of this is often measured with bladder diaries for volume and length between voids.

Pelvic Pain

Chronic pelvic pain (CPP) among women is estimated at a prevalence of around 24% with at least 3 months in length.[19] Patients with CPP have been found to be 3 times more likely to have a history of vaginal delivery, 5 times more likely to report pain with intercourse, and self-reported diagnosis endometriosis or painful cysts.[19] Pelvic girdle instability, abnormal findings with external pelvic/back/abdominal examination, tenderness to palpation of external musculature, and tenderness of the PFM were found among patients with CPP. Women with CPP have been found to have higher levels of serum relaxin.[9] Faulty postural control is also common among women with CPP and consists of increased anterior pelvic tilt leading to lordotic or kyphotic-lordotic postural faults. The abdominal muscles are placed on stretch; thoracolumbar fascia is shortened. Iliopsoas becomes shortened, and hip external rotators shorten.[9] When these factors were addressed in one study, nearly 70% of participants had significant or complete resolution of their CPP.[20]

Physical therapy intervention for CPP should include addressing of the structural and postural deficits with appropriate strengthening and stretching interventions. Symptoms of a nonrelaxing pelvic floor should also be addressed. Nonrelaxing pelvic floor is also associated with voiding dysfunction and sexual dysfunction outside of just pain.[21] Physical therapy intervention may include optimizing lumbopelvic and spinal function, manual therapy (trigger point massage, myofascial release, joint mobilization, and so forth), core stabilization exercises,[21] and behavioral training for bowel and bladder dysfunction.

Biofeedback has been shown to be particularly effective with this population as well in establishing a normal baseline PFM resting tone.[22] Specific interventions will differ based on patient presentation, but in many cases achieving appropriate relaxation of the PFM will include breathing techniques.

Diaphragmatic breathing involves the expansion of the abdominal wall as the diaphragm contracts; given the relationship between the PFM and transverse abdominus activity, the abdominal expansion should translate to PFM expansion as well. This technique is helpful in improving the baseline resting tone but also symptoms associated with voiding[22] and sexual dysfunction when used in these situations.

Dyspareunia

The most commonly cited symptom of CPP is sexual dysfunction and pain with intercourse. The literature frequently reports higher levels of past sexual abuse among this population,[23] and because of this, sexual dysfunction is often a multifaceted problem for patients; it is important to consider a team approach having medical, behavioral, and physical therapy professionals working together. It is also recommended that, although participating in therapy, the patient abstains from intercourse to ensure less pain provocation during the course treatment.

Sexual dysfunction is broken down into 2 categories: superficial and deep dyspareunia. Superficial is most commonly associated with vulvar pain or layer 1 PFM dysfunction.[23] These individuals will often demonstrate a reflexive PFM contraction with sexual penetration or insertion of a digit for assessment. This behavioral change can be addressed with use of self-massage or dilator training[24] to decrease the patient's fear of penetration. Manual therapy is also beneficial in reducing the PFM trigger points and fascial restriction with progressive pressure and stretch applied over the course of treatment.

Deep dyspareunia is often characterized by the presence of muscular trigger points in layer 3 of the PFM, OI, or piriformis. Manual therapy is also notably beneficial here to address muscle restriction, fascial restriction, nerve entrapment, or visceral mobility. These techniques will assist in improving blood flow and vulvar/pelvic mobility. Exercises performed need to focus more on timing, coordination, and the ability to relax over simple contractile strength.[23] Again, a focus on breathing and postural normalization will be helpful in reestablishing an appropriate baseline and decrease reactive/ reflexive contraction in anticipation of pain.

Endometriosis

Endometriosis affects an estimated 10% to 15% of woman in premenopausal years. The condition continues to be a difficult one to manage for the patient and medical professionals alike. Pharmacologic intervention and laparoscopic surgery are well understood as viable treatment options to combat the symptoms and excise visible endometriosis implants, respectively.

There is little agreement in the literature regarding specific physical therapy intervention for treatment of endometriosis. However, many of the side effects of endometriosis can be addressed. Improving the coordination and function of the PFM, addressing scar tissue or adhesions in the pelvis and abdomen, addressing bowel and bladder dysfunction, and improving fascia/visceral mobility can all aid in decreasing the pain associated with endometriosis.[25]

Central sensitization is also common among these patients and down training of the central nervous system may be beneficial in reducing their overall pain. Techniques may include guided imagery, meditation, yoga, breath work, and/or general relaxation training.

Pudendal Neuralgia

Entrapment or injury to the pudendal nerve has been shown in the literature to have wide variations in prevalence. The discrepancy is thought to be a result of the difficulty in diagnosis and the numerous different causes for the resulting pain. Neural entrapment or injury can occur at any one of the points of vulnerability (**Fig. 5**): sacral nerve root, at the sacrospinous ligament, Alcock's canal, where it branches near the ischial tuberosity, or at the distal nerve endings throughout the pelvic floor and perineum.

In women, the most common causes are surgical injury, pelvic trauma, and childbirth.[26] Aside from mechanical injury, nerve irritation can result from noxious stimuli from myofascial, skin, or visceral pain.[27] This visceral pain should be first ruled out to ensure an underlying pathologic condition is not driving the pain. Once completed, a thorough examination of the PFM and associated structures by a PT will determine if shortened muscles, trigger points, or fascial restriction is leading to the nerve irritation. If unsuccessful, then nerve conduction studies and possible nerve block may be warranted. These patients tend to fall into the category of chronic pain and will present with central sensitization, meaning that

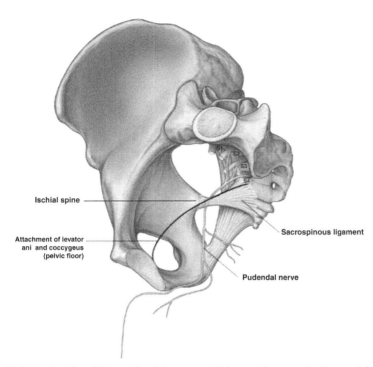

Ischial spine

Attachment of levator
ani and coccygeus
(pelvic floor)

Sacrospinous ligament

Pudendal nerve

Fig. 5. Unilateral path of the pudendal nerve as it leaves the sacral spine and branches to the perineum. (*From* Drake RL, Vogl AW, Mitchell A. Pelvis and perineum. In: Gray's anatomy for students. 3rd edition. Elsevier: Philadelphia; 2015. p. 437; with permission.)

pharmacologic and/or surgical intervention may not be sufficient to help them overcome their symptoms.

All too often, however, the physical therapy evaluation is put off in lieu of other medical interventions, and the musculoskeletal dysfunction that may be underlying goes untreated. A biomechanical screen, evaluation of the connective tissue, examination of the internal and external pelvic musculature, and assessment of neural tension are valuable for the proper understanding of the patient's condition.[27] Treatment with manual therapy, education on the condition, PFM, and general relaxation training, and home exercise program for strengthening and stretching should be used to ensure normalization of tone and release of entrapment. The length of treatment of pudendal neuralgia can vary greatly so the patient should be prepared for the possibility of slow recovery based on the mechanism of injury or chronicity of the condition.

SUMMARY

Physical therapy has many benefits and is a less-invasive and well-tolerated supplement to traditional medical interventions for obstetric and gynecologic patients. Understanding the role that these practitioners can play in the recovery and treatment process can be a valuable addition to the patient's team of allies. Prevention and early intervention through a PT can be effective in reducing the patient's risk for many of the diagnoses discussed.

REFERENCES

1. Anatomy manual: Pelvis. 1997. Available at: http://www.emory.edu/home/index. html; http://www.emory.edu/ANATOMY/AnatomyManual/pelvis.html. Accessed October 14, 2017.
2. Vleeming A, Stoeckart R, Snijders C. The sacrotuberous ligament: a conceptual approach to its dynamic role in stabilizing the sacroiliac joint. Clin Biomech 1989; 4:210–3.
3. Mahakkanukrauh P, Surin P, Vaidhayakarn P. Anatomical study of the pudendal nerve adjacent to the sacrospinous ligament. Clin Anat 2005;3:200–5.
4. Kegel A. Sexual functions of the pubococcygeal muscle. West J Surg Obstet Gynecol 1952;10:521–4.
5. Barral JP, Croibier A. Manual therapy for the peripheral nerves. New York: Elsevier; 2007.
6. Laycock J, Haslam J. Therapeutic management of incontinence and pelvic pain: pelvic organ disorders. London: Springer- Verlag; 2002.
7. Mogren I, Pohjanen A. Low back pain and pelvic pain during pregnancy: prevalence and risk factors. Spine 2005;30(8):983–91.
8. Maclennan A, Green R, Nicolson R, et al. Serum relaxin and pelvic pain of pregnancy. Lancet 1989;328(8501):243–5.
9. Baker P. Musculoskeletal origins of chronic pelvic pain: diagnosis and treatment. Obstet Gynecol Clin North Am 1993;20(4):719–42.
10. Stuge B, Laerum E, Kirkesola G, et al. The efficacy of a treatment program focusing on specific stabilizing exercises for pelvic girdle pain after pregnancy. Spine 2004;29(4):351–9.
11. Spitznagle T, Leong F, Van Dillen L. Prevalence of diastasis recti abdominis in a urogynecological patient population. Int Urogynecol J Pelvic Floor Dysfunct 2007; 18(3):321–8.
12. Chiarello C, Falzone L, McCaslin K, et al. The effects of an exercise program on diastasis recti abdominis in pregnant women. J Womens Health Phys Therap 2005;29(1):11–6.
13. Davis D. The discomforts of pregnancy. J Obstet Gynecol Neonatal Nurs 1996; 25(1):73–81.
14. Dietz H. Pelvic floor trauma following vaginal delivery. Curr Opin Obstet Gyencol 2006;18:528–37.
15. Abrams P, Anderson K, Birder L, et al. Fourth international consultation on incontinence recommendations of the international scientific committee: evaluation and treatment of urinary incontinence, pelvic organ prolapse, and fecal incontinence. Neurol Urodyn 2010;29:213–40.
16. Jarvis S, Hallam T, Lujic S, et al. Peri-operative physiotherapy improved outcomes for women undergoing incontinence and or prolapse surgery: results of a randomized controlled trial. Aust N Z J Obstet Gynaecol 2005;45:300–3.
17. Bø K. Pelvic floor muscle training is effective in treatment of female stress urinary incontinence, but how does it work? Int Urogynecol J Pelvic Floor Dysfunct 2004; 15:76–84.
18. Miller J, Ashton-Miller J, Carchidi L, et al. Does a three-month pelvic muscle exercise intervention improve the effectiveness of the knack in reducing cough induced urine loss on standing stress test? Int Urogynecol J 1998;46(7):870–4.
19. Tu F, Holt J, Gonzales J, et al. Physical therapy evaluation of patients with chronic pelvic pain: a controlled study. Am J Obstet Gynecol 2008;198:272.e1-7.

20. King P, Myers C, Ling F, et al. Musculoskeletal factors in chronic pelvic pain. J Psychom Obstet Gynaecol 1991;12:87–98.
21. Faubion S, Shuster L, Bharucha A. Recognition and management of nonrelaxing pelvic floor dysfunction. May Clin Proc 2012;87(2):187–93.
22. Rao S. Biofeedback therapy for constipation in adults. Best Pract Res Clin Gastroenterol 2011;25(1):159–66.
23. Rosenbaum T, Owens A. The role of pelvic floor therapy in the treatment of pelvic and genital pain-related sexual dysfunction. J Sex Med 2008;5:513–23.
24. Goldfinger C, Pukall C, Gentilcore-Saulnier E, et al. A prospective study of pelvic floor physical therapy: pain and psychosexual outcomes in provoked vestibulodynia. J Sex Med 2009;6:1955–68.
25. Sarrel S. Five things that pelvic health physical therapy can do to improve your endometriosis-related pain. Endometriosis.org global forum for news and information. 2015. Available at: endometriosis.org/news/opinion/five-things-that-pelvic-health-physical-therapy-can-do-to-improve-your-endometriosis-related-pain/. Accessed November 4, 2017.
26. Hibner M, Desai N, Robertson L, et al. Pudendal neuralgia. J Minim Invasive Gynecol 2010;17(2):148–53.
27. Weiss J, Pendergast S. Pitfalls in the effective diagnosis and treatment of pudendal nerve entrapment. Int Pelvic Pain Soc VISION 2006;13(3):1–3.

A Clinician's Approach to the Diagnosis and Management of Recurrent Pregnancy Loss

Deborah A. French, PA-C, MSPAS, MT (ASCP)

KEYWORDS

- Recurrent pregnancy loss • Recurrent miscarriage
- Unexplained recurrent miscarriages • Diagnosis and management
- Controversial treatment

KEY POINTS

- Recurrent pregnancy loss, a condition affecting 1% to 5% of couples, can be challenging for clinicians to manage and devastating to patients needing answers.
- Generally accepted guidelines on the diagnosis and treatment are reviewed.
- More than 50% of patients do not have a diagnosis for the cause of their miscarriages.
- Multiple treatment options have been used for unexplained recurrent miscarriage patients; however, evidence is lacking. Larger clinical trials are needed.

INTRODUCTION

Miscarriage is a devastating event that can occur spontaneously in 15% of all clinically recognized pregnancies.[1] Up to 5% of women of reproductive age, however, experience recurrent pregnancy loss (RPL).[2] Statistics vary in the literature depending on which definition is used for RPL. Classically, RPL has been defined as the loss of 3 or more pregnancies before 20 weeks. Currently, researchers and the American Society for Reproductive Medicine (ASRM) have revised the definition of RPL to 2 or more failed consecutive pregnancies. Although many patients consider they are pregnant based on a home pregnancy test, ASRM defines clinical pregnancy as a pregnancy confirmed by ultrasonography or histopathologic examination.[2] Unfortunately, this definition leaves a lot of gray area, such as a well-documented biochemical pregnancy or a patient who experiences a home miscarriage without previous ultrasound and when the products of conception (POCs) are not examined. On the contrary, the Royal College of Obstetricians and Gynaecologists (RCOG) defines miscarriage as the loss of all pregnancies from the time of conception to 24 weeks, when the fetus would reach viability.[3] This broader definition of pregnancy and miscarriage is more practical

The author declares that she has nothing to disclose.
Advanced Internal Medicine, University of Kentucky, 2605 Kentucky Avenue #402, Paducah, KY 42003, USA
E-mail address: French731@gmail.com

Physician Assist Clin 3 (2018) 457–468
https://doi.org/10.1016/j.cpha.2018.02.012   physicianassistant.theclinics.com
2405-7991/18/© 2018 Elsevier Inc. All rights reserved.

in the clinical setting when supporting grieving patients with a positive pregnancy test that did not result in a live birth.

The diagnosis and management of RPL can be both challenging and frustrating because there are both generally accepted and controversial etiologies and treatments. The controversy stems from the lack of large clinical trials, conflicting studies, or little to no evidence in the literature. Despite this deficit in evidence, well-intending clinicians continue to focus on theoretic etiologies and unproved treatments, which can lead to misleading results.[4] Unfortunately, 50% of RPL patients do not have a clear diagnosis despite a full work-up,[5] leaving clinicians and patients desperate for answers and treatment options. The goal of this article is, first, to review etiologies that have been associated with RPL and the recommended and controversial evaluation and management. Second, this article gives clinicians a proposed approach for the diagnosis and management of patients with this intimidating disorder.

RISK FACTORS AND MANAGEMENT OF RECURRENT PREGNANCY LOSS
Anatomic Etiologies

Uterine anomalies, both congenital and acquired, can account for up to 19% of RPLs.[6] Most commonly, congenital anomalies lead to second-trimester pregnancy loss. It is a debate on the role uterine malformations play in first-trimester RPLs but the assessment of the uterine cavity is generally recommended. Congenital uterine anomalies that potentially cause RPL include unicornuate, didelphic, bicornuate, septate, and arcuate uteri.[2] Due to the vascular insufficiency, septate uterus is the most common of the anomalies, causing up to 35% of RPLs.[7] Acquired anomalies that may contribute to RPL include fibroids, endometrial polyps, and uterine adhesions. The management of these issues, however, in regard to RPL is controversial. Uterine fibroids are the most common of the defects that are acquired, but their role in RPL and management is debatable and may depend on size and location to determine if surgical management is warranted. A majority of uterine anomalies can be detected in the office using saline infused 3-D ultrasound, which is also the most cost-effective test for evaluating the uterus. Other diagnostic studies performed outside of the office can include hysterosalpingogram, hysteroscopy, laparoscopy, and MRI.

It is the general consensus that surgical correction in patients with RPL who have significant uterine cavity defects should be considered. Particularly, in cases of women with RPL and septate defects, surgical correction may have some benefit although large randomized controlled studies are lacking.[2] The role of fibroids and RPL is not completely understood, but it has been stated that submucosal fibroids should be surgically removed when diagnosed in these women to increase pregnancy potential.[8]

Genetic Etiologies

After 2 or 3 miscarriages, a genetic evaluation of the POCs and the parents should be considered early in the work-up. In couples with RPL, 3% to 5% have chromosomal abnormalities in 1 of the partners. Of these patients, the most common chromosomal anomaly associated with RPL is a balanced translocation,[9] a chromosomal anomaly in which there is an exchange of genetic material between chromosomes. Even though this is a small portion of RPL patients, this information can be the key in determining appropriate next steps and to give patients realistic expectations.

The most common cause of pregnancy loss at less than 10 weeks is embryonic aneuploidy. Cytogenic abnormalities account for at least 50% of all miscarriages. In couples with RPL, chromosomal anomalies occurred in the POCs 30% to 57% of the time.[10] Obtaining a karyotype of either the POC or the parents can be costly but should not be undervalued because it plays a key role in further investigations. After obtaining a karyotype of the POC, it may only be necessary to obtain a karyotype of the parents if a chromosomal anomaly was found in the embryo or fetus.[11]

If a chromosomal defect has been identified, it is important to refer to genetic counseling. Another proposed treatment is in vitro fertilization with pregenetic screening or pregenetic diagnosis. The procedure entails removing a cell from the embryo, screen or test for a specific genetic abnormality, and only transfer embryos that do not have the defect. Although studies have shown a decrease in the miscarriage rate with pregenetic screening or pregenetic diagnosis, the live birth rate was higher in couples with chromosomal anomalies who naturally conceived.[12] This option is not for everyone due to the expense and stress of a failed in vitro fertilization cycle, but the literature suggests that these couples may still have a high probability of a live birth without treatment. Using donor gametes may also be a viable option in cases of embryonic aneuploidy that is almost inevitable.

Antiphospholipid Syndrome

Antiphospholipid syndrome (APS) is generally known as a cause of RPL and is considered the most important treatable cause.[12] The presence of antiphospholipid (aPL) antibodies has been identified in 5% to 20% of patients with RPL and is part of the diagnostic criteria for APS.[2] In a systematic review of 5270 women, it was concluded that a woman with 1 or more of aPL antibodies has a 3-fold higher risk of pregnancy failure.[13] In addition to RPL, APS has also been associated with preeclampsia with multiple studies showing moderate to high levels of aPL antibodies in women with severe preeclampsia.[14]

A diagnosis of APS requires the presence of 1 clinical and 1 laboratory criteria. Complete diagnostic criteria are outlined in **Fig. 1**. Testing of APS is only recommended in patients who meet the clinical and laboratory criteria, which include a history of venous thrombosis and/or pregnancy morbidity and a positive lupus anticoagulant, anticardiolipin antibodies, or anti-β_2 glycoprotein.

With the exception of these specific laboratory tests, "other clinical assays associated with APS are not standardized, therefore, not recommended."[2]

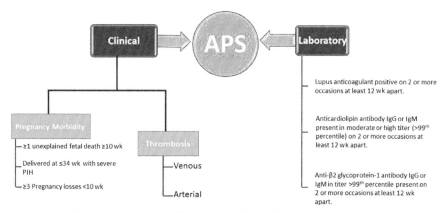

Fig. 1. International consensus classification for APS. Patients should have at least 1 clinical and 1 laboratory criteria sometime in the course of their disease. PIH, pregnancy-induced hypertension. (*Data from* Refs.[9,14,15])

Multiple treatment options have been used, including aspirin, heparin, steroids, and intravenous immunoglobulin. Only the combination of unfractionated heparin and aspirin, however, has shown evidence of improved live birth rate in women with APS and RPL.[12] Also, low-molecular-weight heparin (LMWH) has not established comparable efficacy to substitute.[2] Studies on prednisone and RPL did not show improved live birth rates.[2]

Endocrine Factors

Diabetes mellitus

It is known that women with uncontrolled diabetes are at risk of sporadic miscarriage and malformations, but the role in RPL has not been proved higher than the general population.[3] Women with a glycosylated hemoglobin A_{1C} (HbA_{1C}) of greater than 8% have been associated with increased risk of miscarriage but well-controlled diabetes has shown no increased risk.[16] Therefore, a standard diabetes evaluation with HbA_{1C} and or glucose tolerance testing should be performed. Once diagnosed with diabetes, reaching good glycemic control may reduce the chances of miscarriage. Evidence shows a link with obesity and insulin resistance also increasing the risk of miscarriage. Although it can be a difficult subject to discuss with patients, offering guidance in weight reduction can improve their outcome Although metformin has insufficient evidence on its effects on RPL, it may be reasonable to prescribe this to recurrent miscarriage patients with insulin resistance.[9]

Thyroid antibodies and dysfunction

Thyroid dysfunction has been associated with infertility and poor obstetric outcomes but its role in RPL has not been proved. It has been advised to correct this dysfunction prior to pregnancy. Some researchers suggest that thyroid-stimulating hormone (TSH) levels should be less than 2.5 mIU/L to be considered normal, even though the normal reference range for TSH is much broader.[2] The treatment and the role of subclinical hypothyroidism are, however, controversial. Some studies have shown an association with thyroid antibodies and RPL and a decreased miscarriage rate after treatment, but sufficient evidence is lacking.[17] Laboratory evaluation, including TSH and thyroid peroxidase antibodies, should be obtained in RPL.[14]

Hyperprolactinemia

Hyperprolactinemia is a known cause of infertility and miscarriage. One small randomized controlled trial found a connection between hyperprolactinemia and RPL. It suggests that elevated serum prolactin levels have a negative effect on the corpus luteum, effecting the progesterone levels that sustain early pregnancy. The study found that treating with bromocriptine lowered miscarriage rates and improved birth rates of 85.7% more than 52.4%.[2,18]

Unexplained Recurrent Pregnancy Loss

Despite the efforts of a complete evaluation, 50% to 75% of couples with RPL do not have an explainable cause for their miscarriages.[2] After a full evaluation, including karyotype POC, parental karyotype, and anatomic, endocrine, and autoimmune causes that have been ruled out, a patient is considered as having unexplained RPL. Before diagnosing the patient, the POC should consistently have a normal karyotype, and lifestyle factors associated with miscarriage should be addressed and corrected.[11] It is also important to address maternal age and the number of prior miscarriages with unexplained RPL to give couples an accurate prognosis. Studies have shown in these patients that the chance of a live birth after 2 years was 70% in women with 3 miscarriages whereas only a 45% chance of live birth in women with 6 miscarriages. Women who were 40 years old only had a 40% chance of live birth in 2 years, whereas women age 30 had a live birth rate of 75%.[11]

Multiple interventions have been suggested for unexplained RPL to improve birth rates, but no effective treatment has been identified.[19] Out of desperation to help these couples, a wide variety of unproved or controversial therapies have been used by clinicians. One study, using a combination of rednisolone, 20 mg/d × 12 weeks; progesterone 20 mg/d ×12 weeks; aspirin, 100 mg/d until 38 weeks; and folate, 5 mg every second day throughout the pregnancy, suggested a higher birth rate in comparison to no treatment of women with RPL. Live birth rates in the treatment group were 72% and 35% in the control.[20] The significance is questionable, however, due to the small sample size of 52 in each group.

It is repeatedly stated in the literature that women with unexplained RPL have an excellent prognosis in achieving a live birth without the need of surgical or pharmacologic intervention. In addition, the RCOG advises that the use of empirical treatment in these women is "unnecessary and should be resisted."[3] Furthermore, within the literature, several studies have suggested the concept of psychological support in regard to improving live birth rates. There are no specific guidelines as to what constitutes psychological support, but in general it involves close obstetric care in subsequent pregnancies. Brezina and Kutteh[9] created an environment of support that begins immediately after a pregnancy is diagnosed. The patients are monitored closely, starting with evaluation of quantitative human chorionic gonadotropin levels at least twice and evaluation of appropriate progesterone levels. An early transvaginal ultrasound is scheduled and it is advised to relay encouraging signs of a progressing pregnancy. The ultrasound is repeated in 1 week, again relaying encouraging results. In women with RPL, the presence of a normal heart rate in the developing embryo in 2 consecutive ultrasounds between 6 weeks and 8 weeks has shown a live birth rate of 82%.[9,21] Conveying these statistical results to RPL patients can provide them with some of psychological support they need.

Psychological Factors

Miscarriage can have a huge psychological effect on couples and it is advised that clinicians be sensitive to this during follow-up evaluations and during future pregnancies. Patient with RPL tend to have anger depression, anxiety, grief, and guilt.[2] It has been suggested that there could be a link to psychological factors and miscarriage. Studies have shown a significant improvement in pregnancy outcomes with close monitoring and support at a dedicated RPL clinic in subsequent pregnancies.[2]

Lifestyle and Environmental Factors

After the initial shock of a miscarriage, couples often want to know if it was something they did wrong or an exposure that caused the pregnancy loss. It is important to let them know that exercise, intercourse, and diet do not cause miscarriages[9] and that more than half of all miscarriages occur as a result of a chromosomal abnormality[10] that they could not prevent. Clinicians should focus on factors that have a connection with miscarriage and counsel on the correction or elimination.

Caffeine

Several studies have shown a correlation of increased risk of miscarriage with caffeine in excess of 300 mg per day, the equivalent of 2 cups of coffee.[9]

Smoking

Cigarette smoking is known to decrease fertility and increases the risk of miscarriage. The etiology is suggested that smoking has an adverse effect on trophoblastic function.[2]

Alcohol consumption
Drinking 2 or more alcoholic beverages a week during pregnancy can increase the risk for first-trimester miscarriage.[22] In addition, when combined with other negative habits, such as smoking in the same individual, there is a 4-fold increased risk.[9]

Obesity
Obesity has been defined as a body mass index of greater than 30 kg/m² and has an association with increasing the risk of miscarriage.[9]

CONTROVERSIAL TOPICS
Inherited Thrombotic Disorders

Pregnancy itself is known to be a hypercoagulable state. Additionally, thrombophilias are responsible for more than 50% of maternal venous thromboembolisms during pregnancy.[23] Theoretically, the relationship between thrombophilias and RPL is based on impaired placental development and function due to a venous or arterial thrombosis leading to miscarriage.[1] Inherited thrombophilias, including factor V Leiden, protein C deficiency, protein S deficiency, prothrombin gene mutation, and antithrombin, may have a relationship with second-trimester and third-trimester losses but has not been proved to cause first trimester RPL. Therefore, it is not recommended to test routinely and only recommended in cases with patients who had a personal or family history of a thrombotic event[24] (**Table 1**).

The treatment of women with inherited thrombophilias and RPL is controversial and more definitive data are needed from controlled clinical trials. Different views exist on the treatment of these patients with aspirin, unfractionated heparin or LMWH, or aspirin and heparin. Although LMWH has shown some benefit in several trials, others have questioned the efficacy of LMWH.[26] Even if studies have failed to show proved benefit of LMWH in RPL patients with inherited thrombophilias, it should always be considered to treat these patients prophylactically for the prevention of thrombotic events throughout reproductive age.[27]

Table 1 Recommended evaluations for inherited thrombophilias		
Test	**Normal Range**	**Note**
Factor V Leiden screening with activated protein C resistance	<2.0	Second-generation coagulation assay[9]
Factor V Leiden gene mutation	Negative	Cost effective to reserve testing when factor V Leiden screening is abnormal[9]
Prothrombin G20210A gene mutation	Negative	PCR testing[9]
Antithrombin activity	75%–130%	
Protein S activity	60%–145%	Free and total protein S antigen levels have been suggested to aid in the diagnosis of protein S deficiency in addition to protein S activity.[25]
Protein C activity	75%–150%	Some cases of protein C deficiency may have normal protein C antigen levels; therefore, protein C activity should be used to diagnose protein C deficiency.[25]

Testing only recommended with a personal or family history of thrombotic event (ASRM Practice Committee 2012)[1].
Data from Refs.[9,25]

Maternal Age

It has been widely accepted that aneuploidy is the most common cause for RPL in women with advanced maternal age due to the increased number of aneuploidy oocytes. The age of the woman affects her probability of RPL. It has been estimated that a woman who is 25 has a theoretic RPL rate of 1.2% and a woman over 45 may exceed 50%.[28] A study looking at basal follicle-stimulating hormone (FSH) levels in unexplained RPL patients failed to show any difference in comparison to controls in women under 40.[28] It has been suggested, however, that rising FSH levels in RPL correlate with a worsened prognosis.[29] Although it is not routinely recommended to test a day 3 FSH level, it may be useful in the counseling of patients over the age of 35.[9]

Autoimmune Factors

An autoimmune response occurs when there is a failure to control normal mechanisms that prevent the immune system from attacking itself. Autoantibodies to phospholipids, thyroid antigens, nuclear antigens, and multiple other autoimmune antibodies have been investigated as possible causes for RPL. There is still controversy, however, over routine testing, which antibodies to test, and treatment in regard to RPL. Women who have both aPL antibodies and systemic lupus erythematosus have been shown to have an increased risk for miscarriage in comparison with those with systemic lupus erythematous and negative aPL antibodies.[30] On the contrary, antinuclear antibodies have not been linked with RPL. Treatment of antinuclear antibodies has been with use of corticosteroids; however, this has been shown to have maternal and fetal complications and does not benefit live birth rates. Therefore, the testing or treatment is not recommended.[9]

Luteal Phase Defect

It has been proposed that a luteal phase defect (LPD) can be a cause of miscarriage and RPL.[17] This is defined as a deficiency in endogenous progesterone causing a negative effect on the endometrium in the luteal phase, which is important for implantation.[17] Inadequate progesterone production from the ovaries can have an impact on early pregnancy.[14] Diagnosing a luteal phase deficiency has been long debated and difficult. Measuring histologic and/or biochemical testing for endometrial dating has been unreliable and not reproducible.[31] Currently, it is not recommended to perform routine endometrial biopsies for investigative purposes for RPL.[2]

Some researchers have advocated for the measurement of serum progesterone during luteal phase to diagnose LPD. If the luteal progesterone level is less than 10 ng/mL, it is abnormal. There has been a lack of correlation, however, between endometrial histology and serum progesterone.[9]

Overall, there is no consensus on the standard management of LPD. The use of progesterone in sporadic miscarriages has been ineffective, but in cases of 3 or more consecutive miscarriages, progesterone supplementation may be beneficial.[2,18,32]

Infection

Multiple infectious agents have been linked to sporadic pregnancy loss, including *Mycoplasma hominis*, *Ureaplasma urealyticum*, and *Chlamydia trachomatis*. Multiple other organisms have also been identified but not seen as frequently. None of the infections, however, has been associated with RPL. Because it is associated with miscarriage, many clinicians obtain cultures in women with RPL and treat both partners.[9] Currently, it is not recommended to do routine cultures in patients with RPL who are asymptomatic or to use antibiotics prophylactically.[2]

Male Factor

Typically, semen parameters are evaluated in the setting of infertility. Recently, studies have focused on sperm aneuploidy and DNA fragmentation, which may be caused by advanced paternal age, environmental factors, toxic exposures, excessive heat to the testicles, and varicoceles.[2] Studies have been contradictory on sperm aneuploidy and the association of RPL; therefore, semen analysis testing is not currently recommended routinely.[2,14]

WORK-UP AND MANAGEMENT

The work-up and management of RPL can be a challenge when comparing evidence-based versus controversial topics that have conflicting data or lack of studies. With the exception of APS, all etiologies or treatment of RPL seem to have debatable topics. The ASRM has stated, regarding the literature on evaluation and treatment of RPL, "these publications do not support definitive conclusions about the causes of RPL." It also goes on to say, "our understanding in this field is in flux."[2] If most topics in the area of RPL are up for debate, how can clinicians give these patients the most comprehensive evidence-based care?

An Algorithm Proposed in Clinical Reproductive Medicine and Surgery

Clinical Reproductive Medicine and Surgery: A Practical Guide, Third Edition,[33] gives clinicians a simplified and clearer approach to the initial evaluation and management for early RPL using the most current evidence. In **Fig. 2**, the initial evaluation for RPL begins after the second miscarriage and starts with the evaluation of fetal POCs. These results determine if further work-up is needed at that point. If the POCs show an aneuploid fetal karyotype, then no further work-up is necessary at that time unless other clinical factors have deemed it necessary. A large portion of these aneuploid embryos are the result of advanced maternal age and the patient should be counseled on future risk of miscarriage. If the POCs show unbalanced chromosome translocation or inversion, it is advised to perform parental karyotypes. These patients should be offered genetic counseling and given the option of preimplantation genetic diagnosis. If the POCs show a euploid karyotype, the RPL work-up should proceed.[33] The further work-up of early RPL is continued in **Fig. 3**. The evaluation begins after 2 miscarriages with either no evaluation or euploid POC. First, it is suggested that the woman has a hysterosalpingogram or sonohysterogram, a saline-infused transvaginal ultrasound that can further evaluate the endometrium for distortions. Surgical treatment may be offered for correction. Next, the algorithm advises an endocrine evaluation, including TSH, prolactin, progesterone, and HbA$_{1C}$. Management targets the specific disorder. The author advises microbiologic evaluation, including a culture and/or endometrial biopsy, even though this has been a topic of debate and not routinely advised.[2] If there is a positive culture, however, the appropriate antibiotics are advised. After 2 miscarriages, most investigators agree that lupus anticoagulant, β_2 glycoprotein 1, and aPL antibodies should be part of the work-up and treated as appropriate. It is also advised to take a good history evaluating for lifestyle or environmental elements that may cause miscarriages. Last, it is appropriate after 2 losses to get a karyotype on each parent and refer to genetic counseling. Pregenetic diagnosis may be appropriate in some cases of abnormal parental karyotypes.

DISCUSSION

Caring for RPL patients can be a daunting task when patients may be angry, depressed, or anxious. With lack of clear guidelines, diagnosing these patients can be intimidating

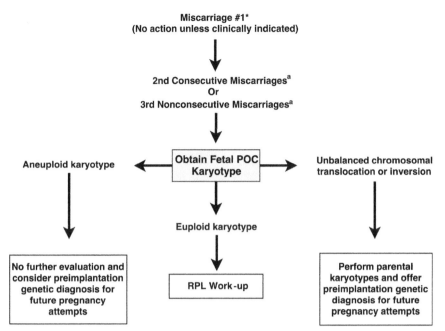

Fig. 2. Initial evaluation for early RPL. An algorithm for the initial evaluation of early RPL. Arrows are provided that guide readers through various outcomes possible during the RPL evaluation and appropriate next steps in diagnostic management. [a] Miscarriage is defined by the loss of a clinical pregnancy documented by ultrasonography or histopathological examination. (*Adapted from* Brezina PR, Kutteh WH. Classic and cutting-edge strategies for the management of early pregnancy loss. Obstet Gynecol Clin North Am 2014;41:1–18; with permission.)

but can be more simplified with the algorithms cited in this article. Treatment of RPL should be aimed at the cause. It is the responsibility of the health care provider to give balanced, evidence-based counseling on options available. Full evaluation should include efforts to rule out identifiable contributing disorders, such as diabetes or thyroid disease, and managing these disorders appropriately. Despite the full evaluation, 50% of patients with RPL do not have a diagnosis after work-up. These patients are diagnosed with unexplained RPL after taking into account age and miscarriage history. Supplementing with progesterone after 3 miscarriages is the only pharmacologic treatment that may have some benefit for unexplained RPL patients. Treatment of unexplained RPL is mainly aimed at modifying lifestyle and environmental factors that may cause miscarriage. In addition, psychological support seems to be the focus with these patients. Brezina and Kutteh[9] have stated that explanation and emotional support are the most important parts of therapy. It is widely stated in the literature that most of unexplained RPL patients have a good prognosis for eventually achieving a successful pregnancy without any treatment other than psychological support.

Many of the etiologies and management of RPL are not in agreement among researchers and are controversial. As a clinician, it is hard to sift through the literature containing many conflicting results, when the main focus is to find something that will work for these patients. Several studies that were performed on this subject showed evidence of sporadic miscarriage, but the evidence for RPL is lacking. Future research looks promising in many different aspects of RPL, but many are still in the experimental phase.

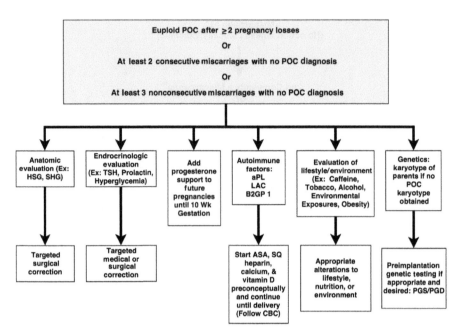

Fig. 3. Work-up for early RPL. An algorithm for the full work-up of early RPL. Arrows are provided that guide readers through various outcomes possible during the RPL evaluation and appropriate next steps in diagnostic and therapeutic management. Not included in this decision tree are more controversial types of testing and therapies, such as those dealing with microbiologic factors, thrombophilic factors, immunotherapy, and other evaluations though these may be appropriate in certain clinical situations. aPL, antiphospholipid; ASA, acetylsalicylic acid (aspirin); B2GP, beta-2-glycoprotein; CBC, complete blood count; HSG, hysterosalpingogram; LAC, lupus anticoagulant; PGS, pregenetic screening; PGD, pregenetic diagnosis; POC, products of conception; SGH, sonohysterogram; SQ, subcutaneous; TSH, thyroid stimulating hormone. (*Adapted from* Brezina PR, Kutteh WH. Classic and cutting-edge strategies for the management of early pregnancy loss. Obstet Gynecol Clin North Am 2014;41:1–18; with permission.)

For now, the ASRM 2012[1] committee opinion and RCOG 2011[3] Green-top Guideline are the most comprehensive evidence-based guidelines to follow.

REFERENCES

1. Evaluation and treatment of recurrent pregnancy loss: a committee opinion. Fertil Steril 2012;98(5):1103–11.
2. Ford HB, Schust DJ. Recurrent pregnancy loss: etiology, diagnosis, and therapy. Rev Obstet Gynecol 2009;2(2):76–83.
3. The investigation and treatment of couples with recurrent first-trimester and second-trimester miscarriage. Green-top Guideline. 2011. 17. Available at: http://www.dcdutta.com/pdf/GTG17recurrentmiscarriage.pdf. Accessed November 30, 2017.
4. Kaiser J, Branch DW. Recurrent pregnancy loss: generally accepted causes and their management. Clin Obstet Gynecol 2016;59(3):464–73.
5. Management of recurrent early pregnancy loss. ACOG practice bulletin. Int J Gynaecol Obstet 2002;78(2):179–90.
6. Jaslow C, Carney J, Kutteh W. Diagnostic factors identified in 1020 women with two versus three or more recurrent pregnancy losses. Fertil Steril 2010;93(4):1234–43.

7. Saravelos S, Cocksedge K, Li T. Prevalence and diagnosis of congenital uterine anomalies in women with reproductive failure: a critical appraisal. Hum Reprod Update 2008;14(5):415–29.
8. Jaslow C. Uterine factors. Obstet Gynecol Clin North Am 2014;41(1):57–86.
9. Brezina P, Kutteh W. Classic and cutting-edge strategies for the management of early pregnancy loss. Obstet Gynecol Clin North Am 2014;41(1):1–18.
10. Fritz B, Hallermann C, Olert J, et al. Cytogenetic analyses of culture failures by comparative genomic hybridisation (CGH)–Re-evaluation of chromosome aberration rates in early spontaneous abortions. Eur J Hum Genet 2001;9(7): 539–47.
11. Kutteh W. Novel strategies for the management of recurrent pregnancy loss. Semin Reprod Med 2015;33(03):161–8.
12. Rai R, Regan L. Recurrent miscarriage. Lancet 2006;368(9535):601–11.
13. Di Nisio M, Rutjes A, Ferrante N, et al. Thrombophilia and outcomes of assisted reproduction technologies: a systematic review and meta-analysis. Blood 2011; 118(10):2670–8.
14. Shahine L, Lathi R. Recurrent pregnancy loss. Obstet Gynecol Clin North Am 2015;42(1):117–34.
15. Wilson W, Gharavi A, Koike T, et al. International consensus statement on preliminary classification criteria for definite antiphospholipid syndrome: report of an International workshop. Arthritis Rheum 1999;42(7):1309–11.
16. Niekerk ECV, Siebert I, Kruger TF. An evidence-based approach to recurrent pregnancy loss. S Afr J Obstet Gynaecol 2013;19(3):61.
17. Hachem HE, Crepaux V, May-Panloup P, et al. Recurrent pregnancy loss: current perspectives. Int J Womens Health 2017;9:331–45.
18. Hirahara F, Andoh N, Sawai K, et al. Hyperprolactinemic recurrent miscarriage and results of randomized bromocriptine treatment trials. Fertil Steril 1998; 70(2):246–52.
19. Ahmed DFUA, Faryad DN. Idiopathic recurrent miscarriages; use of aspirin alone or heparin and aspirin: emperical or evidence based management. Prof Med J 2016;23(09):1033–8.
20. Tempfer CB, Kurz C, Bentz E-K, et al. A combination treatment of prednisone, aspirin, folate, and progesterone in women with idiopathic recurrent miscarriage: a matched-pair study. Fertil Steril 2006;86(1):145–8.
21. Hyer JS, Fong S, Kutteh WH. Predictive value of the presence of an embryonic heartbeat for live birth: Comparison of women with and without recurrent pregnancy loss. Fertil Steril 2004;82(5):1369–73.
22. Gardella JR, Iii JAH. Environmental toxins associated with recurrent pregnancy loss. Semin Reprod Med 2000;18(04):407–24.
23. Lockwood C, Wendel G, Committee on Practice Bulletins—Obstetrics. Practice bulletin no. 124: inherited thrombophilias in pregnancy. Obstet Gynecol 2011; 118(3):730–40.
24. Committee on Practice Bulletins—Obstetrics, American College of Obstetricians and Gynecologists. Practice bulletin no. 132: antiphospholipid syndrome. Obstet Gynecol 2012;120(6):1514–21.
25. Schick P, Schick B. Hereditary and acquired hypercoagulability. 2016. Available at: https://emedicine.medscape.com/article/211039-workup. Accessed November 30, 2017.
26. Alijotas-Reig J, Garrido-Gimenez C. Current concepts and new trends in the diagnosis and management of recurrent miscarriage. Obstet Gynecol Surv 2013;68(6):445–66.

27. Laskin CA, Spitzer KA, Clark CA, et al. Low molecular weight heparin and aspirin for recurrent pregnancy loss: results from the randomized, controlled HepASA trial. J Rheumatol 2009;36(2):279–87.
28. Saravelos SH, Regan L. Unexplained recurrent pregnancy loss. Obstet Gynecol Clin 2014;41(1):157–66.
29. Hofmann G, Khoury J, Thie J. Recurrent pregnancy loss and diminished ovarian reserve. Fertil Steril 2000;74(6):1192–5.
30. Kutteh W, Lyda E, Abraham S, et al. Association of anticardiolipin antibodies and pregnancy loss in women with systemic lupus erythematosus. **Presented at the 40th Annual Meeting of the Society for Gynecologic Investigation, Toronto, Ontario, Canada, March 31 to April 3, 1993. Fertil Steril 1993;60(3):449–55.
31. Murray MJ, Meyer WR, Zaino RJ, et al. A critical analysis of the accuracy, reproducibility, and clinical utility of histologic endometrial dating in fertile women. Fertil Steril 2004;81(5):1333–43.
32. Oates-Whitehead R, Haas D, Carrier J. Progestogen for preventing miscarriage. Cochrane Database Syst Rev 2003;(4):CD003511.
33. Brezina PR, Kutteh WH. Recurrent early pregnancy loss. In: Tommaso F, Hurd WW, editors. Clinical reproductive medicine and surgery: a practical guide. 3rd edition. New York: Springer; 2017. p. 271–88.

Moving?

Make sure your subscription moves with you!

To notify us of your new address, find your **Clinics Account Number** (located on your mailing label above your name), and contact customer service at:

Email: journalscustomerservice-usa@elsevier.com

800-654-2452 (subscribers in the U.S. & Canada)
314-447-8871 (subscribers outside of the U.S. & Canada)

Fax number: 314-447-8029

Elsevier Health Sciences Division
Subscription Customer Service
3251 Riverport Lane
Maryland Heights, MO 63043

*To ensure uninterrupted delivery of your subscription, please notify us at least 4 weeks in advance of move.

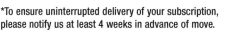